SECOND EDITION

# PUTTING YOUR PATIENTS ON THE PUMP

Karen M. Bolderman, RD, LDN, CDE

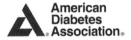

American Diabetes Association.

*Director, Book Publishing,* Abe Ogden; *Managing Editor,* Greg Guthrie; *Acquisitions Editor,* Victor Van Beuren; *Editor,* Rebekah Renshaw; *Production Manager,* Melissa Sprott; *Composition,* Circle Graphics; *Cover Design,* Jody Billert; *Printer,* United Book Press, Inc.

Printed in the United States of America
1 3 5 7 9 10 8 6 4 2

The suggestions and information contained in this publication are generally consistent with the Clinical Practice Recommendations and other policies of the American Diabetes Association, but they do not represent the policy or position of the Association or any of its boards or committees. Reasonable steps have been taken to ensure the accuracy of the information presented. However, the American Diabetes Association cannot ensure the safety or efficacy of any product or service described in this publication. Individuals are advised to consult a physician or other appropriate health care professional before undertaking any diet or exercise program or taking any medication referred to in this publication. Professionals must use and apply their own professional judgment, experience, and training and should not rely solely on the information contained in this publication before prescribing any diet, exercise, or medication. The American Diabetes Association—its officers, directors, employees, volunteers, and members—assumes no responsibility or liability for personal or other injury, loss, or damage that may result from the suggestions or information in this publication.

∞ The paper in this publication meets the requirements of the ANSI Standard Z39.48-1992 (permanence of paper).

ADA titles may be purchased for business or promotional use or for special sales. To purchase more than 50 copies of this book at a discount, or for custom editions of this book with your logo, contact the American Diabetes Association at the address below, at booksales@diabetes.org, or by calling 703-299-2046.

American Diabetes Association
1701 North Beauregard Street
Alexandria, Virginia 22311

DOI: 10.2337/9781580404976

**Library of Congress Cataloging-in-Publication Data**
Putting your patients on the pump / Karen M. Bolderman, editor. -- 2nd ed.
     p. ; cm.
  Rev. ed. of: Putting your patients on the pump / Karen M. Bolderman. c2002.
  Includes bibliographical references and index.
  ISBN 978-1-58040-497-6 (alk. paper)
  I. Bolderman, Karen M., 1954- II. Bolderman, Karen M., 1954- Putting your patients on the pump. III. American Diabetes Association.
  [DNLM: 1. Diabetes Mellitus, Type 1--drug therapy. 2. Insulin Infusion Systems. 3. Insulin--therapeutic use. 4. Patient Education as Topic. WK 820]
  616.4'62061--dc23
                    2012049593.

# Table of Contents

*Acknowledgments* . . . . vii

*Foreword* . . . . ix

*Introduction* . . . . xi

**CHAPTER 1**
**Insulin Pump Therapy Advantages
and Disadvantages** . . . . 1
   Benefits . . . . 2
   Myths . . . . 4
   Challenges . . . . 5

**CHAPTER 2**
**Pump and Infusion Set Options
and Selection** . . . . 9
WITH SUSAN L. BARLOW, RD, CDE
   Pump Features . . . . 9
   Insulin Pump Options and Selection . . . . 10
   Infusion Set and Tubing Options . . . . 16
   Customer Service and Other Practical
      Considerations . . . . 20

## CHAPTER 3

## Pump Candidate Basics . . . . 23

Profile of an Appropriate Candidate . . . . 23

Contraindications: Red Flags . . . . 27

Steps for Helping the Patient Determine and Achieve Readiness . . . . 28

Are YOU Ready? . . . . 30

## CHAPTER 4

## Getting the Patient Ready . . . . 31

Goals and Objectives . . . . 31

Carbohydrate Counting . . . . 35

Hyperglycemia . . . . 37

Hypoglycemia . . . . 38

Infusion Set Insertion . . . . 39

Optional Saline Trial . . . . 41

Lifestyle Issues and Wearing the Pump . . . . 41

Patient Support System . . . . 44

Ordering the Pump and Supplies . . . . 44

## CHAPTER 5

## Pump Start-Up . . . . 47

NICHOLAS B. ARGENTO, MD

KAREN M. BOLDERMAN, RD, LDN, CDE

Pump Start Basics: Patient and Prescriber Responsibilities . . . . 47

Pump Start Guidelines for the Patient . . . . 49

Pump Start Guidelines for the Clinician . . . . 50

Determining Target Blood Glucose Values . . . . 52

Determining Starting Basal Rate . . . . 55

Calculating Insulin-to-Carbohydrate Ratios . . . . 58

Calculating the Correction Factor . . . . 62

Calculating a Meal Bolus . . . . 62

Identifying, Managing, and Preventing Hyperglycemia . . . . 64

Identifying, Managing, and Preventing
    Hypoglycemia . . . . 68
Follow-up Instructions . . . . 69
Additional Considerations . . . . 71

**CHAPTER 6**
# Pump Therapy Management
# (Keeping Patients on the Pump) . . . . 83
Record Keeping . . . . 83
Using Pump Data . . . . 84
Using Blood Glucose Meter Data . . . . 84
Using Continuous Glucose Monitor Data . . . . 85
Basal Rate Adjustment . . . . 86
Additional Basal Rates and Establishing
    Basal Patterns . . . . 89
Temporary Basal Rates . . . . 90
Insulin-to-Carbohydrate Ratio Adjustment . . . . 92
Correction (Sensitivity) Factor Adjustment . . . . 93
Infusion Site and Tubing Concerns . . . . 95
Emergency Supplies . . . . 100
Troubleshooting . . . . 103

**CHAPTER 7**
# Other Considerations in
# Pump Therapy Management . . . . 113
Use of Duration of Insulin Action "Insulin on Board"
    or "Active Insulin" Feature . . . . 113
Dining Out and Special Meals: Bolus Options . . . . 115
Alcohol . . . . 120
Exercise and Physical Activity . . . . 122
    GARY SCHEINER, MS, CDE
Intimacy/Sexual Activity . . . . 129
Managing Sick Days and Medical Procedures . . . . 130
    WITH NICHOLAS B. ARGENTO, MD
Stress . . . . 133
    NICHOLAS B. ARGENTO, MD

Travel . . . . 134
WITH NICHOLAS B. ARGENTO, MD

Weight Change . . . . 140
NICHOLAS B. ARGENTO, MD

Menses, Peri-menopause, and Menopause . . . . 142
NICHOLAS B. ARGENTO, MD

Pregnancy . . . . 142
NICHOLAS B. ARGENTO, MD

Pediatrics: Infants, Toddlers, Children, Teenagers . . . . 146

Type 2 and Type 1.5 (LADA) Diabetes . . . . 158

Older Adults and Special Needs Patients . . . . 162

CHAPTER 8

Forms and Resources . . . . 171

Healthcare Professional Guidelines, Checklists,
and Forms . . . . 171

Patient Guidelines, Checklists, and Forms . . . . 172
WITH NICHOLAS B. ARGENTO, MD

Insulin Pump Therapy Resources . . . . 196
WITH SUSAN L. BARLOW, RD, CDE

CHAPTER 9

Tips from Pump Experts and Case Studies. . . . 203

Tips for Healthcare Professionals from Healthcare
Professionals . . . . 203

Pump Tips for Patients from Patients . . . . 206
WITH SUSAN L. BARLOW, RD, CDE

Case Studies/Success Stories . . . . 219

CHAPTER 10

What Lies Ahead: Insulin Pumps
of the Future . . . . 243
NICHOLAS B. ARGENTO, MD
KAREN M. BOLDERMAN, RD, LDN, CDE

Index . . . . 251

# Acknowledgments

I wanted to be a teacher for as long as I can remember. When I developed diabetes in 1965, my parents, physicians, and teachers encouraged me to learn all that I could about diabetes and to fit diabetes into my life—not build my life around diabetes. Years later, insulin pump therapy made my life with diabetes much easier, and I wanted others to benefit from my experience.

The second edition of *Putting Your Patients on the Pump* would not have been possible without the invaluable contributions of Nicholas B. Argento, MD; Susan L. Barlow, RD, CDE; and Gary Scheiner, MS, CDE. I envisioned this updated version to be a compilation of practical experience and guidance from fellow healthcare professionals who work with pump patients, while living successfully with type 1 diabetes managed with an insulin pump. And that's exactly what I got. Each contributor provided personal and professional information that will benefit healthcare professionals and patients alike. Together with my own personal and professional experience: Dr. Argento's enthusiasm and inclusion of the most current information available, Sue Barlow's expertise and sense of humor, and Gary Scheiner's experience and insightful knowledge, blended together to create a resource to help the novice insulin pump healthcare professional develop confidence implementing pump therapy.

Many people have had an impact on my career as a diabetes educator as well as on my life with diabetes. I am indebted to James (Jim) Mersey, MD,

FACP, FACE, Chief of Endocrinology at Greater Baltimore Medical Center (GBMC) and Medical Director of the Geckle Diabetes and Nutrition Center at GBMC, for providing me with unique and rewarding career opportunities and for teaching me the finer points of diabetes management. Jim's diabetes knowledge, kindness, skillful care for patients, and wisdom are infinite. I am honored that he agreed to write the Foreword to this book.

Maureen D. Passaro, MD, is credited with the idea of the "future" chapter. I also owe much to my former personal physician, G. William Benedict, MD (d, 2006) for his guidance and patience in putting me on my first pump many years ago. And to the select group of the many other patients and physicians who influenced my decision to begin pump therapy and help others make the same decision, I would also like to acknowledge: Riccardo Calafiore, MD; Richard E. Berger, MD, FACP, FACE; and John P. Comstock, MD. I am also thankful to Frank Weller (d, 1997); Scott Fischell; Cindy Shump, RN, MS, MSN, CRNP, CDE; Amy Mersey, RN; Zoe (Heineman) Myers, MA; James A. Dicke, MD; Joanna B. Tyzack, MD; Fran R. Cogen, MD, CDE; Ruth S. Horowitz, MD; and Philip A. Levin, MD, for their dedication and contributions to the field of diabetes and insulin pump therapy.

A special thank you goes out to the reviewers Davida Kruger, MSN, APRN, CDE; Joan Hill, RD, CDE; and Dr. James H. Mersey for kindly providing their time and expertise.

I want to thank the American Diabetes Association for providing me with the opportunity to write the second edition of this book. I am especially indebted to Victor Van Beuren, Acquisitions Editor, for his patience, wisdom, and unending support, and book editor Rebekah Renshaw for her dedicated editorial work and insight.

I extend gratitude also to my loving, very smart, and very patient husband Tom and my extraordinary parents. Additionally, I thank my dear siblings and their spouses, nephews, and nieces for their constant support and encouragement. Thanks also to my professional colleagues through my years as a pump therapy diabetes educator. I am indebted to the countless pump patients with whom I have had the privilege and pleasure to work with and learn from. Their contribution to my knowledge of diabetes has been of untold value, for which I am most grateful.

***Karen M. Bolderman, RD, LDN, CDE***

# Foreword

I have been an endocrinologist involved in the management of diabetes for the past 35 years. I began before glucose meters existed. In 1977 when I started the Diabetes Clinic at The Johns Hopkins University School of Medicine, Ames gave me the first Dextrometer to use. It took several minutes to get a reading on a dial the size of a bathroom scale, but this device signified a huge step forward in diabetes monitoring. When insulin pumps became clinically available, I actively championed their use, although the early ones were the size of an Uzi.

Over the years, pump technology has progressed at a steady pace, with the addition of new ways to deliver insulin, better integration with meters either as built in or by infrared communication, and with use of continuous glucose sensors. All of this brings the hope of a true closed-loop system.

In spite of these improvements in technology, selecting patients for pumps and starting patients on pumps still requires a great deal of education, training, and time, along with knowledge on the part of the healthcare provider.

I have known Karen Bolderman since she began working for me as a diabetes educator 30 years ago. After several years, Karen and I began working together again at the Geckle Diabetes and Nutrition Center at Greater Baltimore Medical Center, where we are working to integrate diabetes care in and out of the hospital.

For us this is déjà vu all over again. We work together to teach patients about pumps, get them started, and manage their diabetes post initiation. With Karen's knowledge and personal experience, starting and training patients on pumps, managing patients in the hospital, and following patients on pumps makes my life much easier. I look forward to a continued partnership with Karen in our attempts to improve diabetes care.

Karen has done a marvelous job with the details of insulin pumps in this edition of *Putting Your Patient on the Pump*. This book will make everyone's job of utilizing insulin pumps more understandable and practicable.

Read ahead and enjoy.

**James H. Mersey, MD**
Director, Endocrinology and Metabolism,
Medical Director, Geckle Diabetes and Nutrition Center
Greater Baltimore Medical Center
Assistant Professor of Medicine,
The Johns Hopkins University School of Medicine
Clinical Associate Professor of Medicine,
University of Maryland School of Medicine,
Baltimore, Maryland

# Introduction

nsulin pump therapy gives people with diabetes the freedom to enjoy life, despite their chronic condition. The value and importance of having freedom are obvious from the impact this innovative technology has made in the past several decades. The insulin pump is now a common, integral component of diabetes management. Technological improvements and advances have made the insulin pump a desirable and useful tool in the management of diabetes.

As long-term insulin pump wearers with type 1 diabetes and healthcare professionals who have learned much from our colleagues and countless other "pumpers," the contributors to the second edition of *Putting Your Patients on the Pump* have a unique perspective and understanding of what constitutes practical, useful information. Collectively, the four of us have lived with type 1 diabetes for over 165 years. Most of these years have been spent with an insulin pump. It is our hope that this book will help healthcare professionals with expertise in diabetes care and education successfully start and maintain diabetes patients on insulin pump therapy. We believe that even experienced clinicians will find the information, tips, and resources helpful.

We hope this book provides user-friendly information from our combined practical experience and supports the extra efforts diabetes healthcare professionals must make to help their patients achieve success using an insulin pump.

*Karen M. Bolderman, RD, LDN, CDE*

## CHAPTER 1

# Insulin Pump Therapy Advantages and Disadvantages

KAREN M. BOLDERMAN, RD, LDN, CDE

Insulin pump therapy is in its fifth decade and is gaining wider popularity. In the U.S., an estimated 20–30% of patients with type 1 diabetes and <1% of insulin-treated patients with type 2 diabetes use an insulin pump (HSBC Global Research 2005). As of this writing, the most current data indicate that there are over 375,000 patients with type 1 diabetes (up from approximately 130,000 in 2002) now using an insulin pump (U.S. Food and Drug Administration, General Hospital and Personal Use Medical Devices Panel 2010). Insulin pump therapy requires fewer "injections" compared with multiple daily injection (MDI) therapy; an infusion site is changed every 2–3 days, for an average of about 152 infusion site insertions/year, while MDI therapy results in about 1,460 injections/year (based on 4/day). Until research yields a practical way to replace lost β-cell function in diabetes, the insulin pump provides the most elegant method of insulin replacement. In its best application, pump therapy is a rare win–win situation in diabetes in terms of glycemic control and personal freedom.

An insulin pump is a wonderful diabetes management tool, but as with any tool, the pump is only as good as the patient's ability to use it. Clinicians have a responsibility to carefully screen and provide access to educational resources to all patients who express an interest in pump therapy. When patients are

**Insulin pump:** A small, programmable, battery-powered device worn externally that delivers insulin in tiny continuous amounts (basal doses) and in larger amounts for meals or hyperglycemia (bolus doses). The pump is attached to the patient by either an infusion set consisting of long, thin flexible tubing with a catheter (or needle) on the end that is inserted subcutaneously into the patient, OR, a tubing-free ("patch") pump is directly attached to the patient with a subcutaneous needle-inserted catheter and self-adhesive tape. The user programs and operates the pump or the pump's remote control device to deliver insulin doses that match individual needs. An insulin pump does not automatically calculate the amount of insulin needed; patients and healthcare professionals work together to calculate the patient's daily insulin amounts, and the pump is then programmed by the patient to deliver insulin based on the person's specific requirements.

mismatched with the pump or the pump regimen, loss of control may occur and potential benefits are lost or nullified.

Successful pump therapy is more likely with motivated and conscientious patients. Regardless of what many patients first think, the pump patient must perform frequent self-monitoring of blood glucose (SMBG), learn how to use their data, and understand how to use their insulin pump to ensure proper pump function and improve or achieve desired glucose control (American Diabetes Association 2004). Also, the patient must calculate food-related bolus insulin doses based on individualized insulin-to-carbohydrate ratios as well as bolus doses to decrease hyperglycemia based on individualized insulin correction (sensitivity) factors.

# Benefits

## For People with Type 1 Diabetes

- Improves glycemic control by delivering an individualized basal rate supplemented with bolus doses to match the patient's intake and correct any hyperglycemia. Erratic glucose fluctuations can potentially be reduced.

- Offers precise dosage delivery in basal rates as low as 0.025 units/h and bolus doses in exact whole, tenth, and twentieth-unit doses.
- Can manage the dawn phenomenon by delivering a higher basal rate during the dawn hours.
- Can control glucose during and after exercise by delivering a lower basal rate.
- Has the potential to decrease the risk of hypoglycemia by allowing patients to individualize insulin doses to match their requirements hour by hour.
- May lessen or reverse hypoglycemia unawareness by decreasing the incidence of hypoglycemia.
- Allows incremental, precise doses to match growth spurts in children and adolescents and to manage people who are insulin sensitive.
- Improves management of patients with gastroparesis by adding the option of splitting and/or extending bolus delivery over time to match delayed absorption of nutrients.
- Can match delayed gastric emptying observed with the use of pramlintide, or with the consumption of high-fat foods, by extending bolus delivery over time.
- Eliminates the frequency and inconvenience of multiple daily injections (MDI).
- Increases lifestyle flexibility by allowing the person to eat at desired intervals instead of matching food intake to injection therapy insulin peak times.
- Improves well-being and quality of life by providing freedom in school, work, exercise, and leisure-time schedule variations.
- Allows for easier weight loss. With individualized dosing, the pump patient is not "chasing insulin" with additional food. Additionally, with decreased incidence of hypoglycemia, caloric intake to treat hypoglycemia is reduced.

## For People with Type 2 Diabetes

- Allows the attainment and maintenance of improved glycemic control
- Eliminates the frequency and inconvenience of MDI.
- Increases lifestyle flexibility by allowing the person to eat at desired intervals instead of matching food intake to injection therapy insulin peak times.

■ Improves well-being and quality of life by providing freedom in school, work, exercise, and leisure-time schedule variations.

■ Allows for easier weight loss. With individualized dosing, the pump patient is not "chasing insulin" with additional food. Additionally, with the potential decreased incidence of hypoglycemia, caloric intake to treat hypoglycemia is reduced.

## For Women Who Are Pregnant or Planning Pregnancy

■ Mimics normal physiology with individualized precise dosage delivery.

■ Has the potential to decrease pre- and postprandial glucose (PPG) excursions.

■ May potentially reduce the risk of hypoglycemia.

■ Improves the management of morning sickness by eliminating the need to eat on rising: a correctly calculated basal rate maintains euglycemia.

■ Allows for easier achievement of recommended blood glucose goals.

■ May potentially reduce postprandial hyperglycemia due to the delayed. gastric emptying of normal pregnancy as well as gastropathy with the use of the extended or combination bolus feature.

# Myths

| Patient | Healthcare Professional |
| --- | --- |
| The pump calculates and delivers all my insulin doses automatically | The pump calculates all the required insulin doses automatically |
| No more SMBG | Any patient can use a pump |
| Can eat whenever I want without planning | Less emphasis on meal planning |
| Can eat as much as I want | Not useful in type 2 diabetes |
| Too expensive | Too expensive |
| Too much trouble | Too complicated for most people |
| Can't wear it during exercise, swimming, or intimacy | Can't wear it during exercise, swimming, or intimacy |

| Patient | Healthcare Professional |
|---|---|
| Can eliminate low and high glucose levels | Can eliminate low and high glucose levels |
| I can lose weight quickly by skipping meals | Will cause weight gain because most patients will start eating more, since they only have to press a button to deliver insulin instead of taking injections |
| Children won't like wearing a pump | Too risky for children to use |
| Can learn how to use a pump in just a few minutes, since I'm very tech-savvy | A pump company representative gets the patient ready and calculates the patient's starting basal rate(s), insulin-to-carbohydrate ratio(s) (ICR), blood glucose goals, and correction (sensitivity) factor(s) as part of the pump training |

The pre-pump and ongoing education and skills training in pump use provided by the healthcare professional are crucial in correcting any misconceptions the patient may have about pump therapy and, even more important, in guiding the patient as s/he develops pump skills. The truth about pump therapy is that the greater the patient's effort and the greater the support and access to skills training, the greater the chance that therapy will succeed. Healthcare professionals as well as patients need to understand the implications of pump therapy, including both benefits and challenges.

# Challenges

Pump therapy is not without some challenges and risks, although a patient with motivation, pre-pump training, and ongoing pump education can tackle practically any drawback. However, inattention to problems can create life-threatening circumstances. Weigh these challenges and risks against the benefits.

- In putting a patient on a pump, there are challenges and risks for the healthcare professional (HCP) as well. Preparing the patient for pump therapy requires an assessment of the patient's "readiness" and diabetes knowledge and coordination of efforts on the part of the patient, pump manufacturer, and diabetes educators. The HCP's initial learning curve, i.e., willingness to learn pump therapy, and the time investment for patient follow-up and management are crucial factors in assuring success with pump therapy.

■ **A learning curve.** Pump therapy requires education, skills training, and initial intensive follow-up and management. A patient contemplating pump therapy must know beforehand how to count carbohydrate and match insulin doses with carbohydrate intake and basal needs. A patient must also know his/her correction (sensitivity) factor(s) and how and when to use a corrective insulin dose. The pump wearer must learn the technical "buttonology" of their specific pump and learn how to insert the battery(ies), fill (if appropriate) and insert the insulin cartridge/reservoir, change the infusion set and tubing (if applicable), and calculate appropriate insulin bolus doses. Intensive follow-up for the first few weeks after pump initiation is essential and includes detailed recordkeeping of glucose levels, carbohydrate intake, exercise, and insulin doses. For children, the learning curve also involves their parents and caregivers.

■ **Frequent SMBG.** The pump wearer must perform a minimum of four glucose checks daily, with additional checks as needed between meals; during sleep hours; before, during, and after exercise; during illness and at times of stress; and when glucose levels become erratic or "unexplainable." Bolus doses of insulin must be calculated to match the person's food intake, anticipated activity, current glucose level, and insulin "on board" from a previous bolus dose(s).

■ **Possible weight gain.** Insulin pumps offer precise dosage delivery to match the patient's food intake. It can become easy for the pump wearer to bolus extra insulin for additional calories. People may begin to eat foods that may have been considered "forbidden" before using a pump and may over indulge in high-calorie foods of low nutrient value. Although glycemic control can be maintained with additional insulin doses for excessive caloric intake, weight gain can result.

■ **Hypoglycemia.** If the basal rates are not set correctly or if the pump wearer miscalculates and overdoses a bolus delivery or doesn't compensate for exercise or for the insulin "on board" from a previous bolus dose(s), hypoglycemia can result. Pattern management is very important.

- **Unexpected hyperglycemia.** If the patient miscalculates or improperly sets the basal rate(s) or bolus doses, hyperglycemia can occur unexpectedly. The rare pump failure or occasional site occlusion or site "blockage" due to overuse and resultant scar tissue can decrease or prevent basal/bolus delivery, resulting in hyperglycemia.

- **Ketoacidosis.** In addition to the potential improper setting of the basal rate(s), the omission of filling the tubing (if applicable), and omission or miscalculation of a bolus dose, the rare pump malfunction may also cause partial or total interruption in the basal delivery. Because the pump uses only rapid-acting insulin, there is no "background" insulin available for hyperglycemia and the prevention of ketonemia. However, studies from the past three decades revealed a decrease in diabetic ketoacidosis in pump wearers compared with patients using MDI therapies (Bruttomesso 2009).

- **Skin irritation and infusion site infections.** People with sensitive skin may develop redness, tenderness, itching, or rashes from the infusion set or pump self-adhesive tape. Those who perspire heavily or participate in water sports may have problems with getting the tape to stick to their skin. Removing the adhesive may also cause concern. Site infections can occur from poor insertion technique or leaving the infusion set or pump (if applicable) in place too long.

- **Logistics/placement.** Although the insulin pump weighs about 4 oz and is smaller than a smart phone, wearing it creates challenges. Despite offering flexibility in lifestyle, many people may find it unpleasant or intolerable to be connected 24 h a day to a small external device. Pumps that use tubing to connect to an infusion set require a clip, a case with a built-in clip, or a belt-loop case for attachment. Some people prefer to place their pump in a pocket, whereas others may choose to wear their pump discreetly under clothing. Tubeless or patch pumps cannot be moved into pockets. They can be placed under clothing, but when wearing or changing clothes that do not cover or "hide" them (such as sleeveless tops or low-waisted slacks), because the pump's adhesive is applied to the skin, the pump is immovable until the infusion set and site are changed several days later. Intimacy/sexual activity, showering or bathing, exercise, and contact sports create additional challenges in how to wear the pump.

■ **Medical requirements.** Some insurance companies may require that a potential pump patient provide SMBG records and/or a medical necessity form completed by the healthcare professional, as well as certain lab reports (such as recent A1C or C-peptide levels) before the patient is "approved" for the purchase of an insulin pump.

■ **Paying for it.** In 2013, the average price of an insulin pump is between $6,000 and $8,000. Disposable supplies, including pump batteries, insulin cartridges/reservoirs, infusion sets, and skin preparation products can add up to an additional $1,500 or more per year. As of this writing, a recent introduction to the pump market offers a lower initial "setup" cost but requires disposable components that may cost slightly more than standard pump supplies, thus enabling the disposable components to be covered under a patient's insurance for supplies rather than durable medical equipment. In general, increased insurance reimbursement for pump therapy has helped to increase its use (Scheiner 2009). Some insurance companies cover all or some of the expense, whereas others may provide for only the pump and not the supplies, or vice versa. Advise your patient to be thoroughly familiar with the costs before making a commitment to pursue pump therapy. Pump manufacturers are happy to work with a potential pump patient's insurance company to investigate coverage and out-of-pocket costs.

## REFERENCES

American Diabetes Association: Continuous subcutaneous insulin infusion (Position Statement). *Diabetes Care* 27(Suppl. 1):S110, 2004

Bruttomesso D, Costa S, Baritussio A: Continuous subcutaneous insulin infusion (CSII) 30 years later: still the best option for insulin therapy. *Diabet Metab Res Rev* 25:99–111, 2009

HSBC Global Research: Diabetes: proprietary survey on insulin pumps and continuous blood glucose monitoring. Healthcare U.S. Equipment & Supplies, 2005

Scheiner G, Sobel RJ, Smithe DE, Pick AJ, Kruger D, King J, Green K: Insulin pump therapy: guidelines for successful outcomes. *The Diabetes Educator* 35(Suppl. 2):29S–43S, 2009

U.S. Food and Drug Administration, General Hospital and Personal Use Medical Devices Panel: Insulin Infusion Pumps Panel Information, 2010

## CHAPTER 2

# Pump and Infusion Set Options and Selection

KAREN M. BOLDERMAN, RD, LDN, CDE
SUSAN L. BARLOW, RD, CDE

## Pump Features

Several manufacturers sell insulin pumps and infusion sets. A pump company may offer more than one model. Each pump has slightly different features. And there are many different types of infusion sets available for pumps that are connected to the patient with an infusion set (versus a "patch/pod/tubeless" pump).

What kind of pump—standard with tubing and infusion set or "patch"/pod? A pump that is totally "contained," or one that has a disposable component to it? The latter style pump's settings are programmed into the "hardware" part of the pump and the section of the pump containing a pre-filled insulin cartridge is connected to the main component section, used for several days (with tubing attached to the person's body), removed, and replaced, thus saving on the initial financial investment. There are many different pump brands and models to choose from.

Most pumps connect to the body via tubing of various lengths and an infusion set. A patch/pod or "tubeless" pump system consists of an integrated glucose meter and remote control device to operate the insulin "pod," which is attached to the skin similarly to an insulin infusion set with self-adhesive tape. An insulin pod is a combination of an insulin pump cartridge/reservoir and infusion set. The patient fills the pod with the amount of insulin to be infused over several days and attaches the pod via the built-in cannula. A patch/pod pump eliminates the need for tubing, as the infusion set and pod holding the insulin are an integrated system. The pod delivers the insulin using the remote control device that is programmed with the user's pump settings, such as basal rates, bolus options, etc. Some models provide the option of delivering a bolus directly from the pod.

After 2–3 days' use, the pod is disconnected from the skin and discarded, and replaced with a new pod that the pumper again fills with the appropriate amount of insulin. A pod is shaped similarly to a small half hard-cooked egg and is attached to the body with self-adhesive tape. Once in place, it is not "moveable," as there is no tubing. Patch or "pod"-style pumps provide another option in pump therapy without the "hassle" factor of tubing. Many people prefer the freedom that a tubeless pump allows, while other people may not like the "immovable lump" appearance of the patch pump and might prefer to "move the pump around" and wear it outside or inside clothing. Of course, pod placement can be as discreet as wearing a tubing-style pump under the clothing.

# Insulin Pump Options and Selection

Experience with one brand of pump may bias a physician or educator toward that pump even when another brand or model may suit the patient as well, or better. Sometimes clinicians assume that their personal preferences for pump features are the same as the patient's. As much as possible, allow the patient to choose their pump. Remember that you are preparing and managing the patient's pump therapy, NOT training the patient on the "buttonology" or button-pushing aspects of the pump. Don't allow your personal pump brand choice, bias, or comfort level with a particular brand dictate the pump the patient chooses. The patient's preference is paramount and can be a factor in successful implementation of pump therapy.

Deciding on a suitable choice usually takes time. Give the patient enough time to read the marketing literature, surf the various pumps' websites (some have "virtual" interactive pumps to simulate use/practice), view the various pump manufacturer DVDs, review diabetes publications comparison lists and articles about pumps, and meet with the pump manufacturer sales representatives and/or clinical staff. As the prescribing clinician, if you have been provided with several manufacturers' "demo pumps," offer to demonstrate several pumps to the patient. This may be helpful after the patient has done some research and is able to discuss features that appeal to them. Remember that, like all cars that get you from one place to another, all pumps deliver insulin but vary in their colors, options, features, and degree of sophistication.

## Pump Criteria Checklist
### General

Is the pump a patch/pod type, eliminating the need to be "connected" to infusion set tubing 24/7 but requiring a remote device or wireless device/meter combination for all programming?

Does the pump have advanced programming features that would be used for "fine-tuning" basal and bolus delivery and be implemented over time? Some pumps are sophisticated or "smart" and have options for fine-tuning insulin, while other pumps offer basic basal–bolus features that may be more appropriate for a person with type 2 diabetes who would not use the sophisticated, more advanced "smart pump" features.

- Ease of navigating on-screen selections (user "friendliness" or intuitive use) Does the pump utilize touch-screen technology and/or have minimal button pressing and scrolling?
- Is the pump screen easily visible? Does it have color and/or contrast making it easy to see and operate under a variety of light conditions?
- Use of icons, words, or abbreviations (and color)
- How much memorization is required? Is it difficult to remember how to move from one screen or function to another?
- For a child, could someone only slightly familiar with the pump (caregiver, teacher, babysitter) stop it or perform troubleshooting? Is there a lock feature and/or remote control?
- Ease of manual tasks: Could a user with hand arthritis, carpal tunnel syndrome, or neuropathy use the pump easily?
- Does the user need to fill the cartridge/reservoir with insulin or does the pump use brand-specific pre-filled cartridges? Are there many steps in "loading" the cartridge/reservoir into the pump?
- How many steps are involved in changing or entering a program?
- Can the pump user choose between hearing audible sounds and alarms (in varying sound volumes) and a vibratory mode for all pump functions?

- How long does the battery(ies) last? Are batteries easy to obtain and replace? Does the pump require charging and how often? How easy is it to replace a lost charger or obtain a back-up charger?
- Does the pump have a specific infusion site/set change reminder alert or alarm that can be programmed to sound or vibrate at a time chosen by the user every 2–3 days (or as determined appropriate) to serve as the reminder to change the infusion set/site? This is one of the most useful features ever designed for insulin pumps. A "general" or non-specific alarm that can be set for whatever reason the pump user decides is not nearly as useful. The importance of changing the infusion site/set often cannot be stressed enough to new as well as experienced pumpers.
- What type of clock is available, 12-h or 24-h? Does the pump have the option for both 12-h and 24-h? This is important, as patients who use the 12-h clock may inadvertently switch AM to PM and deliver the wrong basal doses throughout the day. Downloaded history may not alert the patient to this error. Most pumps today offer both clock options, but basal rates are most accurately programmed using the 24-h clock.
- Does the pump have multi-language capacity?
- What is involved in detaching the pump?
- Does the pump have a backlight? How long does the backlight stay lit, and is the duration of time adjustable?
- Is the pump waterproof or watertight? Does it require any special accessories to make it waterproof? This is a consideration not just for water sports, as daily activities also expose the pump to water, such as accidentally dropping the pump into the toilet or using it in the shower/bath.
- What is the size of the pump? How thin is the pump? Can it be worn discreetly under clothing?
- How much does the pump weigh?
- Does the pump have the option of using a remote device for all its programming and delivery functions?
- Is there an audio, vibrate, or remote option for patients who want to wear the pump discreetly?
- How is a patch/pod/tubeless pump attached to the person? How strong is the adhesive? Can the pod be temporarily disconnected?
- How is a standard pump with tubing worn/attached to the person? Are there options, including a removable clip, a case with a built-in clip, a case

with built-in belt loops, or a choice of other cases? Is the case available in a variety of colors and materials (leather, vinyl, plastic, etc.)? Do case options include something like a "skin" used on cell phones to provide a grip and ease in holding the pump? Will the pump fit into a "universal" case, i.e., one that accommodates various pumps so that the patient may be able to purchase a case from another pump manufacturer?

- Is the pump available in more than one color? If not, can the user change the outside color or appearance of the pump?
- With what device can the pump communicate? Most insulin pumps can wirelessly communicate with either a blood glucose (BG) meter or a continuous glucose monitor (CGM). As of this writing, interconnectivity among all three devices is not yet available, but the integration of these technologies is on the horizon. Determine what is most important for the patient—the ease of wireless transmission of the BG from the meter to the pump for calculation of insulin doses, or use of a CGM device.
- What types of history does the pump store? Percentage of total daily dose (TDD) as basal and as bolus? Most recent boluses? A summary of daily delivery, including TDD, an average of TDD over X number of days, amounts of insulin delivered as correction boluses and meal boluses, infusion set changes? Total history, including alarms, alerts, battery changes, infusion set changes, and basal rate/pattern changes?
- Does the pump include software to download data reports of various types that can be used by both the patient and healthcare professional to track trends, make changes and corrections, and monitor overall use of the pump?

## Insulin and insulin delivery

- What size is the cartridge/reservoir, i.e., how much insulin can it hold? Does the pump use a disposable cartridge/reservoir, or is the cartridge "built into" the pump? How much insulin can the cartridge/reservoir hold? This varies, and as of this writing ranges from 176 units to 315 units. This is important for people who are insulin resistant or use large doses of insulin. Remember that tubing connects the cartridge/reservoir to the infusion set and the tubing must be primed (filled) with insulin with each infusion set change (see "Sets with tubing," page 97). A set change occurs every 24–72 hours, and the amount of insulin (approximately 20 to 45 units depending on the tubing length) changed/wasted (from discarding the tubing) should be taken into consideration. This may increase overall costs of the insulin supply. Overall, this is an important consideration in choosing a pump whose cartridge/reservoir contains <200 units for use in a patient requiring >55–60 units/day.

■ Some pumps make noise during basal and bolus deliveries. The noise can be a "clicking" or "zzzz-sounding" type noise. Does this matter to the user?

■ Frequent insulin delivery is an important issue for infants, toddlers, children, and insulin-sensitive adults. If the infusion set cannula or metal/steel needle is not infusing insulin constantly, subcutaneous or scar tissue may build up and occlude the site, impeding basal delivery. In contrast to pumps with solenoid motors, a direct-current motor pump delivers fractions of any basal rate, no matter how high or low, in "micro" pulses every 3 minutes. Insulin-sensitive patients are better matched to direct-current motor pumps.

## Basal rate delivery

■ Does the basal rate deliver in increments of 0.10 (tenth of a unit), 0.05 (twentieth of a unit), or 0.025 (fortieth of a unit)? Smaller increments are useful for fine-tuning basal rate delivery in children and insulin-sensitive people.

■ Can the user temporarily increase and decrease basal rate delivery, and for how long? Can the pump be programmed to automatically calculate increases or decreases in percentages for several different basal rates, or can it alternately just calculate the number of units or units/hour? A temporary basal increase is helpful for acute illness or preceding menstruation, whereas a temporary decrease in basal delivery is useful for exercise.

■ How many 24-h basal rate programs can be programmed into the pump? This is useful for patients who want to accommodate activity levels that vary day-to-day. For example, if weekend activity levels are different from weekday activity levels, the user may want to pre-set different 24-h basal programs with higher or lower rates instead of frequently resetting temporary basal rates. The ability to set alternate 24-h basal programs is a helpful feature for children who have gym class on specific days, adults who exercise on alternate days, and patients who are shift workers or weekend athletes, and is also useful for times of premenstrual syndrome, stress, and illness.

## Bolus delivery

■ What types of bolus delivery options does the pump have? Is the bolus delivery increment in twentieths, tenths, halves, or whole-unit increments, or does the user have a choice? Patients who are insulin sensitive may prefer or require fractional-unit bolus increments.

■ Is there more than one type of bolus delivery available? An extended ("square wave") or combination immediate/extended ("dual wave") bolus delivery is useful for patients with gastroparesis and also may be used when consuming high-protein, high-fat, or ethnic meals and if using pramlintide. How long can delivery be extended? Can the delivery be in increments of an hour, such as 15, 30, or 45 minutes?

■ Is there a touch bolus button? Is it audio or vibratory? This is a consideration for the patient who prefers to wear the pump discreetly and does not want to visibly press buttons on the pump or use a remote device to deliver a bolus.

■ Is there a remote device available to deliver a bolus?

■ Can specific bolus types be "named" and programmed into the pump for ease of use, such as "pizza," "ethnic meal," "dessert"? This is helpful and alleviates the need to repeatedly program a frequently used combination ("dual wave") bolus.

■ How is "insulin on board" (active insulin) calculated for bolus deliveries, i.e., can the user determine the number of hours the most recent bolus is active, or does the pump automatically default to a specific duration of time setting, such as 4 hours? This is a useful feature to prevent "insulin stacking" for repeated correction boluses (see page 113). How does the insulin on board feature account for the insulin dose required for the upcoming meal?

■ Does the pump store a history of bolus deliveries? How many? Can this information be downloaded to track trends and patterns of use and dosages?

## Safety

■ Can a bolus dose be stopped easily during delivery? Can the user track exactly how much of the bolus was delivered before it was halted?

■ Is there a maximum use lockout feature for children, so that a basal rate or bolus delivery cannot be programmed for more than a specific upper limit?

■ Is there a time-out feature that the user can pre-set to halt all insulin delivery if a button is not pushed for a specific duration of time?

■ Can the user set an hourly limit of insulin delivery?

■ What type of safety and performance checks does the pump have? How often does the pump perform self-checks?

■ What types of warning and alarm systems does the pump have? Is there an alarm for undelivered basal insulin?

■ Does the pump alarm sound/vibrate when insulin is running low or the cartridge/reservoir is empty? How is the amount indicated? Is it approximate or exact?

■ If batteries are removed for an extended period of time, does the pump retain its memory of programmed basal rates and history of bolus doses and alarms?

■ Is the warning and/or alarm signal visual, auditory, or tactile? If audio, how loud is it? Patients may need a pump with vibrating warnings and alarms.

■ In case of a major technical problem, is a backup pump provided? What are the procedures to obtain a backup pump if one is not provided at the time of purchase? How quickly does the patient receive the replacement pump?

■ What is the repair policy? If the pump is returned for problems, is it repaired and reissued to the patient, or is a new pump provided? Are refurbished pumps redistributed?

# Infusion Set and Tubing Options

Infusion sets distributed by the various pump and pump supply manufacturers may be interchangeable to work with several different brands of pumps or they may be proprietary and brand-specific. Some sets may be designed specifically for a particular age group, such as pediatric. It is best to check with each pump company for specific availability and recommendations and make sure your patient explores all the options with the assistance of the pump manufacturer.

An infusion set is inserted subcutaneously and the set "base" is attached to the insertion site with self-adhesive dressing or tape. An infusion set is worn for 1–3 days and then removed and discarded. Infusion sets left in longer can lead to infection and/or scarring, which slows insulin delivery. Although many brands exist, there are basically two types of infusion sets: metal/steel needle cannula and Teflon cannula, and both types are available in various models. Most infusion sets connect to an insulin pump using a Luer-lock connection, and thus are universal and can be used with a variety of pumps. Advise the potential pumper to be aware of pumps that use a proprietary infusion set, as their choice of infusion sets will be limited unless the pump has an adapter that allows it to accept a Luer-lock infusion set (Roche 2012).

A metal/steel needle infusion set is inserted at a 45- to 90°-angle and requires that the needle stay under the skin. The insertion base and tubing are attached to the site with either self-adhesive or separate dressing or tape. A metal/steel needle infusion set can be disconnected from the infusion site (close to the site or several inches from the site), thus providing lifestyle comfort for physical activity, bathing, and sexual activity. A variety of needles are available by type (straight or bent) and length. Children and lean adults may need shorter needles, and active people may need longer needles to guarantee subcutaneous insertion and placement. A metal/steel needle set may be appropriate for patients who have problems with kinking or dislodgment of Teflon cannula sets. A metal/steel needle set is made of surgical stainless steel and can contain up to 12% nickel and may not be appropriate for people who experience an allergic reaction to nickel or stainless steel (Roche 2012). Some people find the metal/steel needle sets to be uncomfortable because the needle may "pinch" or be felt during physical activity or movement. A metal/steel needle set should be changed every 24 to 48 hours (Roche 2012). A major advantage of the metal/steel needle infusion set is the guarantee of insulin delivery, as a metal/steel needle cannot kink below the skin like a Teflon cannula set. Many parents of child pumpers like them because they are easy to teach to the child's teacher or babysitter in case the child's usual cannula set becomes dislodged. Metal/steel needle infusion sets are also often recommended during pregnancy because they may be easier than a Teflon cannula to insert in the abdominal area or a "hard to reach" (such as the upper hip/buttocal) area and they guarantee insulin delivery with no risk of a kinked or bent cannula.

The metal/steel needle infusion sets had been in use for several decades when pumps were first introduced. They are generally less costly than the soft Teflon cannula sets but are not as commonly used today. Some people choose to alternate use of both types of sets depending on their activity or exercise.

An allergic reaction to the adhesive in the dressing or the glue used to manufacture the infusion sets can occur; trial and error with different products is recommended to determine individual sensitivity.

Because every person can react differently to infusion set material, suggest your patient try a variety of sets. Pump manufacturers and trainers may be able to provide a sample of a few different sets for the patient to try.

A soft Teflon cannula set uses a stainless steel introducer needle that is threaded into the cannula for a 20- to 90°-angle subcutaneous insertion, depending on the brand and the angle of the needle (angled 30 to 45° versus straight 90°). Teflon cannula sets are latex-free and do not contain PVC (polyvinyl chloride). After insertion the needle is removed (having been under the skin just a few seconds), leaving only the cannula below the skin and the infusion set base at the site. The set base has self-adhesive tape or dressing. With a 30°- to 45°-angled set, there is a clear "window" area in the self-adhesive tape, allowing visibility of the site of the catheter insertion. The clear window allows the user to detect the status of the site, including signs of redness or other problems. A 90°-angle set does not have a viewing window, and the user may not be aware of dislodgment or problems until hyperglycemia occurs. Some people find the length of a cannula infusion set introducer needle intimidating and require reassurance and practice in insertion. Some cannula infusion sets have an insertion device to help with insertion (see below). A cannula set can be more comfortable to wear than a metal/steel needle set because the patient cannot feel the set when bending, twisting, or exercising.

Teflon cannula sets may be straight or angled and come in different lengths ranging from 5.5 to 17 mm. The shorter lengths are typically inserted at a 90° angle, while the longer lengths are inserted at a 20 to 45° angle. A short cannula (5.5 or 6 mm) may have a higher failure rate in non-slender adults and probably should not be used initially except in slender patients. And cannula infusion sets come in a variety of models: some are stationary, while others can rotate or change position depending on how the user prefers the tubing to be directed (right or left side, upward or downward). Additionally, some manufacturers offer infusion sets in a choice of colors other than white/clear. New infusion set models are introduced fairly frequently; be aware of the latest available options.

Depending on the brand, a Teflon cannula set can be inserted manually, or with a built-in injector that is disposed after use, or an optional handheld device to facilitate insertion of the needle. Some people prefer the use of an injector system or device, while others may find the clicking noise bothersome. Over time, most patients develop a preferred angle of manual insertion and placement that cannot be determined with the use of an insertion device. Even if your patient chooses to use an insertion device, recommend the patient also learn manual set insertion in case the inserter device is unavailable or becomes lost or broken. No matter what type of infusion set is used, the set should be inserted in one smooth motion (Roche 2012).

Teflon cannula sets can also disconnect at or close to the site, providing lifestyle comfort and flexibility. The user unclips the tubing from the set base, leaving only the base and subcutaneous cannula in place, while removing the tubing and the pump. Some infusion sets may disconnect a few inches from the set base, leaving a short tubing "tail." Some disconnect sets are self-sealing at the time of disconnection, whereas others require covers at the site as well as the end of the tubing.

A Teflon cannula set is more commonly used than a metal/steel infusion set. The latter is an option that you may recommend if your patient experiences problems with Teflon infusion set kinks or dislodgment, but this is not as common as it had been in past decades. Teflon cannula sets must be changed every 48 to 72 hours.

Some infusion sets are packaged with or without tubing, and some are packaged with extra "bases," which allow changing of the metal/steel needle or Teflon cannula every few days, while using the tubing for several days longer, depending on the type of insulin used and other factors (see page 97). The latter type of packaging may be priced less than standard set base/tubing combination packages. Most infusion set combination packages are packaged 10 sets/box.

Discuss the features and benefits of each type of set—metal/steel and Teflon cannula—with your patient. Some patients use both types of sets and alternate depending on their activity.

Infusion set tubing comes in lengths ranging from 18 to 43 inches, depending on the manufacturer and the set. Manufacturers usually offer two or three tubing length options. Some manufacturers offer both clear and colored tubing. The colored tubing may help make it easier for the patient to view the insulin flow and detect air bubbles, which, if large (extending several inches), can account for non-delivery of insulin resulting in unexpected hyperglycemia.

Patients choose tubing length depending on their physical activity, sleeping habits, and clothing. For example, restless sleepers and people who wear their pump in their sock need longer tubing; those who wear the pump at their waist may prefer shorter tubing. Longer tubing may prevent dislodgment of the infusion set when using the bathroom (toilet) while the pump is attached to or in the pockets of pants that have been lowered to the floor. Any excess tubing can be easily tucked into the patient's clothing and kept out of sight and there are companies that make devices that roll up tubing.

Additionally, some infusion sets allow tubing to be "directed," i.e., the tubing position on the base can be changed, depending on the direction preferred by the user (right, left, upward, downward). Tying the tubing in knots does not impede the delivery of insulin, as the tubing is co-extruded (i.e., it has an inner small-diameter tube inside an outer tube). Advise the patient that if s/he would like to try different infusion sets or tubing lengths, their next order can include other available options offered by their pump manufacturer. The same is true for infusion set dressings, as some patients may experience an allergic skin reaction to the self-adhesive tape and may need to try another brand.

# Customer Service and Other Practical Considerations

The pump manufacturer sales personnel should explain the start-to-finish process to both the potential pump user and to his or her healthcare professional or team. The pump patient must be confident that technical support and assistance are available 24 hours a day, 7 days a week. All pumps should have the company's toll-free customer service number displayed on the back of the pump and/or remote device and corresponding communication devices (BG meter, CGM device).

Another consideration is the procedure for ordering supplies. The pump wearer should know what types of infusion sets, accessories, batteries, and specific pump items, such as cartridges/syringes, are needed. Most likely, replacement supplies are obtained by mail order from the pump manufacturer or pump supplier as contracted by the patient's insurance company. Rarely are pump supplies available through a local pharmacy. Some manufacturers or supply companies offer to send the patient supplies routinely and automatically. What role does the manufacturer play in verifying insurance coverage for supplies?

On average, the price of an insulin pump ranges between $6,000 and $8,000, and most come with a 4-year warranty. Some pumps may cost less, as they may have disposable components, thus, less costly "hardware." Medicare currently allows a pump to be replaced every 5 years (DHHS 2013). Supplies, including batteries, pump cartridges/syringes, infusion sets, skin prep items (and other items such as tape/dressing) can cost in excess of $1,500 each year. Help the patient understand the price of both the pump and supplies. Insurance coverage ranges from 50 to 100%, with most averaging about 80% coverage. Some insurance companies may provide coverage for the pump but not the supplies, or vice versa. Some patients have insurance policies with a high deductible or a low cap, such as $500/year, for durable medical equipment or medical supplies, which may be unfeasible for some patients.

The pump manufacturer should give a detailed cost estimate in writing to the patient and keep in touch with the patient throughout the insurance verification and pump and pump supplies ordering process. Usually, a pump manufacturer insurance specialist handles this process. The patient is required to sign an assignment of benefits document, allowing the pump manufacturer to determine the type and amount of insurance coverage provided. This can take one day to several weeks to process. An insulin pump is a prescription item, and the prescribing physician must provide the prescription and/or an order for an insulin pump and corresponding pump supplies to the patient and/or insurance company. Some insurance companies require a letter of medical necessity from the prescribing physician with additional documentation, which may include:

- Several weeks or months of SMBG records
- Recent A1C levels
- Reasons why an insulin pump may be necessary, e.g., erratic glucose pattern correction, preconception, pregnancy, diabetes complications requiring improvement in control, or lifestyle change

Almost every pump manufacturer has a standard "letter of medical necessity" checklist form. An individualized letter from the healthcare professional is rarely required except in the case of an appeal following a pump coverage rejection.

Some insurance providers may allow only certain contracted brands of insulin pumps. The patient should check with their insurance provider to confirm whether or not this is the case before selecting and ordering a pump. Patients who decide on an alternative brand usually need a letter or certificate of medical necessity from the prescribing physician explaining why another pump brand is preferred or required. Because this delays purchase and shipment of the pump, many clinicians have developed form letters to expedite the insurance approval and appeal process. Even if not initially covered, persistence can lead to a non-contract or nonformulary pump approval. Some patients pursue insulin pump insurance coverage for several brands of pumps and opt to settle for the pump that costs the least amount of money. Other patients are firm in their choice and are willing to provide whatever documentation the insurance company may require to approve a noncontract or nonformulary pump.

Patients can often request that the company ship the insulin pump directly to the home. However, overzealous and excited patients have been known to self-initiate pump therapy without formal training and have ended up in the emergency room in DKA or hypoglycemic shock. For this reason, some clinicians and diabetes educators request that the company ship a new pump to their site rather than to the patient's home and insist that pump manufacturers provide scheduled formal pump training. Note that some physicians do not want to accept the liability of having a pump shipped to the office, as there is potential for the pump to be misplaced or lost, or to have it opened inadvertently, or even stolen. For this reason, some pump manufacturers prefer to ship the pump directly to the patient requiring a signature upon delivery. When a pump is shipped directly to the patient, advise the patient to check the shipping list for full contents. Direct the patient to review the pump tutorials and materials prior to office instruction. In either instance, reinforce to the patient to NOT initiate pump therapy without both formal training from the pump manufacturer and the presence of a health-care professional (preferably the pump prescriber or designated HCP).

## REFERENCES

Department of Health and Human Services (DHHS) Centers for Medicare & Medicaid Services: National Coverage Determination (NCD) for Infusion PUMPs (280.14) http://www.cms.gov/medicare-coverage-database/details/nca-details.aspx?NCAId=40&NcaName=Insulin+Infusion+Pump&CoverageSelection=National&KeyWord=insulin+pump&KeyWordLookUp=Title&KeyWordSearchType=And&bc=gAAAABAAAAAA& Accessed 10 February 2013

Roche Insulin Delivery Systems, Inc.: ACCU-CHEK Guide to Infusion Site Management. Fishers, IN: 2012

Scheiner G: Matching patients to devices: diabetes products are not one-size-fits-all. Clinical Diabetes 30:126–129, 2012

## CHAPTER 3

# Pump Candidate Basics

## Profile of an Appropriate Candidate

### Is Your Patient Ready, Willing, and Able?

Many patients are naturals for pump therapy, but it is not for everyone. Some patients need to overcome specific obstacles before the pump will be an asset to their healthcare. Others just do not have the interest or abilities to master pump therapy. Discovering the character and source of motivation through careful screening of the patient is the key to ensuring success in pump therapy.

You must evaluate the physical and psychological readiness of each pump candidate to take on the responsibilities and challenges of pump therapy. The person with diabetes and his or her family need to buy into pump therapy. Input from the patient's family and other members of the healthcare team will help you discern the patient's clinical and lifestyle indications for insulin pump therapy (Table 1).

### A Good Prospect: Ready, Willing, and Able

- **Is motivated.** Pump therapy requires readiness, preparedness, and a time investment for weeks or months in advance and during the initiation of pump therapy.
- **Has realistic expectations.** The patient who expresses interest and desire for pump therapy must understand that the pump will not "fix" blood

glucose variations automatically, nor will pump therapy grant freedom from frequent SMBG. Pump therapy does not guarantee "good control," but it can help achieve and maintain improved glucose control with effort from the pump wearer. Children who use the pump must have parents and caretakers with a thorough understanding of what pump therapy involves and the willingness to spend the time needed working with the child and healthcare professionals.

- **Demonstrates independent diabetes management.** Ideally, MDI therapy precedes pump therapy. MDI as a "stepping stone" to pump therapy often reveals the patient's suitability. At the very minimum, the prospective pump user should have knowledge of the basics of diabetes education. A thorough knowledge of diabetes and its management and the ability to demonstrate appropriate self-care behaviors (including troubleshooting and problem-solving skills) provide the foundation for the advanced self-management skills required by pump users.

| TABLE 1. Indications for Pump Therapy |
| --- |
| **CLINICAL INDICATIONS** |
| Inadequate glycemic control despite optimized MDI therapy |
| High glucose variability |
| Elevated A1C |
| Recurrent, severe, or unpredictable hypoglycemia |
| Nocturnal hypoglycemia |
| Hypoglycemia unawareness |
| Recurrent hyperglycemia |
| Dawn phenomenon |
| Preconception |
| Pregnancy |
| Extreme insulin sensitivity |
| Gastroparesis |
| Early neuropathy or nephropathy, when improvement in glucose control can reduce acceleration of complications |
| Renal transplantation |
| **LIFESTYLE INDICATIONS** |
| Erratic schedule |
| Varied work shifts |
| Frequent travel (probably accompanied by frequent dining out) |
| Desire for flexibility |
| Inconvenience of MDI |

This is one of the reasons pump therapy may not be recommended for newly diagnosed patients (Shalitin 2012).

- **Is willing to learn.** The person must be able and willing to learn, practice, and demonstrate an understanding of carbohydrate counting, insulin action, and premeal bolus dose calculations using their insulin-to-carbohydrate ratio(s) and correction factor(s), and be able to make insulin dose adjustments in response to hypoglycemia, hyperglycemia, exercise, stress, and illness.

- **Has ability to problem-solve.** i.e., can use newly acquired skills in managing diabetes.

- **Welcomes challenges.** The initial few weeks of pump therapy require detailed record keeping of SMBG results, dietary intake, insulin doses, and exercise, as well as frequent (minimum of four daily) blood glucose checks, including "middle of the night" checks (typically at 3:00 a.m.), and frequent (sometimes daily) telephone/email/fax communication with the healthcare professional(s). The pump user must also have patience during the pump initiation period, when appropriate basal rates and insulin-to-carbohydrate ratios are being determined.

- **Has the support of family or significant other(s).** The decision to initiate pump therapy is a lifestyle-changing decision. Emotional support is crucial to the success of pump therapy. Family members, friends, coworkers, teachers, and others can be of great assistance to the pump wearer. Education about diabetes in general, along with pump therapy education, can help ease the difficulties and challenges of pump therapy initiation.

- **Can afford it.** Pumps and pump supplies cost thousands of dollars, so verifying the patient's ability to afford pump therapy is essential. The pump wearer must have either personal resources or adequate insurance benefits. Insurance coverage can range from 50 to 100% for the pump and/or pump supplies. Ask the potential pump wearer to verify their benefits with their health insurance carrier; some pump manufacturers will provide this service to patients. Some insurance companies require a letter of medical necessity from the healthcare prescriber. Additionally, an insurer may cover only a specific brand of pump but may provide benefits for a nonformulary brand with a letter of medical necessity outlining why a specific pump brand (i.e., the pump's features) is most appropriate for the patient. Medicare covers a pump for a patient with type 1 or type 2 diabetes who (A) has completed a comprehensive diabetes education program, performs at least 4 daily SMBG checks, uses at least 3 injections per day, and meets one or more other glycemic control-related criteria; OR (B), if a patient has been on a pump prior to enrollment in Medicare and has documented frequent (minimum of 4 daily) SMBG checks during the month preceding enrollment and meets one or more other glycemic control-related criteria. Additionally, a prospective or current pump patient must have a documented fasting C-peptide level ≤110% of the lower limit of normal of a lab's range (e.g., up to and including 0.99 ng/ml, if the low range is 0.9 ng/ml) or be beta-cell autoantibody positive for Medicare insulin pump coverage. The positive autoantibody test allows patients with latent autoimmune diabetes in adulthood (LADA), referred to as type 1.5 diabetes, to qualify for a pump. Always confirm current Medicare coverage. The pump must be ordered by and follow-up care must be managed by a physician who manages multiple pump patients and who works closely with a team, including CDEs, RDs, and nurses who are knowledgeable in use of pump therapy (DHHS 2013).

■ **Is capable intellectually, physically, and technically.** A patient contemplating pump therapy must be able to demonstrate an understanding of the therapy. Intellectually, the patient must demonstrate understanding of insulin-to-carbohydrate ratios and correction (sensitivity) factors and the applications of these parameters to determine appropriate insulin bolus doses. The ability to insert the pump battery(ies), fill and/or place the insulin cartridge/reservoir into the pump, insert the infusion set, wear the pump, and perform the technical functions of the pump is essential.

- Patients with moderate to severe hand arthritis or neuropathy may not be able to press the pump's buttons or remote device or handle the insulin cartridge/reservoir and infusion sets.
- Patients who are blind or visually impaired may be limited in their choice of pump because of a lack of audio functions or small screen displays.
- Patients who are deaf or hearing impaired may be at greater risk for interruptions in insulin delivery because they have difficulty hearing the pump's alarm. Pumps with vibrating alarms may be essential.

■ **Demonstrates emotional stability.** The pump patient must routinely attend education sessions and attend to tasks that require routine. A patient with untreated depression, eating disorders, manipulative behavior, or other psychoses is usually ill-suited for pump therapy. Carefully assess the pump candidate's psychological status, or refer the patient to a mental health professional. Suggest treatment options for behaviors that may interfere with pump therapy.

Young or old, age in itself is not necessarily a contraindication to successful pump therapy. Children as young as newborns and people in their 70s have had success with pump therapy.

The patient's education level is not a deciding factor in pump therapy. However, diabetes knowledge and an understanding of the relationship between insulin and food, stress, and exercise are key factors in assuring successful pump therapy.

# Contraindications: Red Flags
## Why the Patient Isn't Ready for Pump Therapy

Although pump therapy does not increase the risk of mortality among its users, the frequency of adverse events increases with:

- Poor candidate selection
- Infrequent SMBG
- Insufficient or inadequate supervision and monitoring by the diabetes healthcare professional or team
- Inexperienced pump therapy practitioners

## Indications that the Patient Is Not an Appropriate Candidate

There can be numerous reasons why a patient may not be an appropriate candidate for pump therapy. However, this doesn't mean the patient may not ever be ready for an insulin pump. Behavioral changes, diabetes knowledge, and maturity in dealing with diabetes challenges come with time and education. Be aware that any of the concerns below can be corrected, thus improving the patient's readiness to take on pump therapy:

- Complains of performing frequent blood glucose checks: thinks that pump therapy reduces or omits the need to perform SMBG
- Is "tired of meal planning," counting carbohydrate, and calculating mealtime insulin doses: believes that the pump automatically calculates necessary bolus doses without any user input
- Does not want to carry any "diabetes supplies," e.g., back-up injection device, insulin, hypoglycemia treatment (and when using pump therapy, spare infusion sets)

- Doesn't understand the causes, prevention, and treatment of hypoglycemia
- Is not aware of glucagon and doesn't have a plan for its use (i.e., a family member or significant other trained in the administration of glucagon)
- Doesn't understand the causes, prevention, and treatment of hyperglycemia
- Is not aware of ketone strips, does not have ketone strips, or does not know when/how to check for ketones
- Lives alone and does not have a readily accessible support team (family, friends, coworkers, access to emergency services)
- Has evidence of a psychiatric disorder, including severe or recurrent depression, severe eating disorder, or a history of attempted suicide
- Lacks insurance or means to pay for an insulin pump and pump supplies

# Steps for Helping the Patient Determine and Achieve Readiness

You may be able to identify good candidates for insulin pump therapy, but patients still need to decide whether pump therapy is for them. Here is an education plan for helping the patient make this decision.

1. Give the patient a general overview of what pump therapy entails. Discuss the advantages and challenges, as well as realistic goals and expectations for pump therapy.
2. Review the prospective pump user's medical history and evaluate his or her diabetes knowledge. Consider using written pre- and post-tests.
3. Demonstrate how an insulin pump works (bolus delivery). Explain basic pump therapy terms, including basal rate, bolus dose, infusion set, infusion sites, dressing, and insulin cartridge/reservoir. Show available models, and encourage the patient to learn the features offered by each brand of pump. Explain that he or she can disconnect the pump for bathing, intimacy, and intensive sports.
4. Have the patient handle a pump. Some patients mistakenly believe the pump is worn only during the day and removed at bedtime. Others believe an insulin pump is surgically implanted or permanently attached. Most people are surprised to learn how small a pump is and how it is worn.
5. Show the differences between a pump that uses tubing that connects to an infusion site and a pump that is worn without tubing and is directly connected to the body.

6. Show the available infusion sets. Explain that tubing (if applicable) is available in various lengths to accommodate where the pump is worn. Explain how a pump with tubing can be worn in and under clothing, such as in a pocket, sock, or bra. Show pump accessories, such as clips, leather cases, fanny bag–type cases, clothing with built-in pump pouches or pockets, and Velcro-attached removable pockets or small (infant-sized) socks. Show appropriate sites for wearing a "patch" pump that does not require tubing.

7. Demonstrate the insertion and removal of an infusion set. Demonstrate an infusion set inserter device, if appropriate. Allow the patient to practice a self-insertion. There is a commercially available injection pad, or "rubber belly," that attaches to the patient's abdomen, thigh, or upper arm with an adjustable strap. Does the patient want to wear an infusion set for a few days to get accustomed to the feel of it? If possible, offer the option of wearing a demo pump with saline for a few days to determine how the patient likes that particular pump and pump therapy in general (see Optional Saline Trial, page 41). When parents are considering pump therapy for their child, this experience sometimes results in postponing pump therapy; the parents recognize the learning curve and time commitment a pump requires, or they discover that their child is not quite ready. Because saline is a prescription item, the prescribing physician will need to provide a "saline-start" order and a prescription for saline. Pump manufacturer personnel—either a Certified Pump Trainer or clinical staff—will provide brief training on the pump. Some patients wear two or three brands of pumps before making a final decision.

8. Provide a list of the various pump manufacturers with names and telephone numbers of the local sales representative, corporate office telephone numbers, and website information. Encourage the patient to access pump company websites (monitored by the pump company) and contact the manufacturers' sales representatives, who will offer "sales calls" to patients and/or provide additional information, such as literature and a DVD. Pump company "online pump school" website instructions may also be available. Does your protocol place the responsibility of contacting pump manufacturer sales representatives on you? Is there a local pump support group meeting that the patient can attend to meet pump users and other potential pump patients? Encourage the patient to speak with other pump wearers and potential pumpers via face-to-face conversations or the use of social media.

# Are YOU Ready?

Additionally, the HCP who initiates pump therapy should also consider his/her ability to effectively start and maintain a patient on an insulin pump. Although there are benefits to the patients for insulin pump therapy, there is also the potential for confusion and inadequate training (Skyler 2007), which can create additional work and anxiety for the HCP. An effective and efficient office practice infrastructure is essential. Do you have the time and/or staff to help prepare a potential pump patient and then follow/manage the new pump patient closely the first few weeks after pump initiation (Hirsch 2010)? Ineffective follow-up, likewise, can create problems for the HCP as well as for the new pump patient. Learn about the resources available to you—local Certified Diabetes Educators (CDEs), diabetes centers, and pump company clinical support staff (company-employed or per diem contracted CDEs) can be of great assistance.

## REFERENCES

Department of Health and Human Services (DHHS) Centers for Medicare & Medicaid Services: National Coverage Determination (NCD) for Infusion PUMPs (280.14) http://www.cms.gov/medicare-coverage-database/details/nca-details.aspx?NCAId=40&NcaName=Insulin+Infusion+Pump&CoverageSelection=National&KeyWord=insulin+pump&KeyWordLookUp=Title&KeyWordSearchType=And&bc=gAAAABAAAAAA& Accessed 10 February 2013

Department of Health and Human Services (DHHS) Centers for Medicare & Medicaid Services: Decision Memo for INSULIN Infusion PUMP (CAG-00041N) http://www.cms.gov/medicare-coverage-database/details/nca-decision-memo.aspx?NCAId=40&NcaName=Insulin+Infusion+Pump&CoverageSelection=National&KeyWord=insulin+pump&KeyWordLookUp=Title&KeyWordSearchType=And&bc=gAAAABAAEAAA& Accessed 10 February 2013

Hirsch IB: Practical pearls in insulin pump therapy. *Diabetes Technol Ther* 12 (Suppl 1):S23–S27, 2010

Shalitin S, Lahav-Ritte T, Lebenthal Y, Devries L, Phillip M: Does the timing of insulin pump therapy initiation after type 1 diabetes onset have an impact on glycemic control? *Diabetes Tech Ther* 14:1–9, 2012

Skyler J, Ponder S, Kruger D, Matheson D, Parkin C: Is there a place for insulin pump therapy in your practice? *Clin Diab* 25:50–56, 2007

# Getting the Patient Ready

## Goals and Objectives

It may seem like a simple concept to "get the patient ready" for pump therapy, but as the HCP responsible for prescribing the pump to the patient, it is also your responsibility to make sure the patient is prepared to achieve and maintain success with pump therapy.

Formal training of the patient to use a pump has three stages: prepump education, pump start-up, and pump therapy follow-up and management. Prepump education is usually spread over a few weeks, with a minimum of three visits of 1–3 h each. The usual pump start-up (see Chapter 5) consists of one 3- to 4-h session. Pump follow-up and management can range from a few weeks to several months.

When planning the prepump education, consider both the learning style of each patient as well as their general diabetes knowledge. Some pump patients complete just two to three 1-h preparation sessions with a verbal exchange of information, whereas others need a structured learning situation, such as several 1- to 3-h sessions or classes spread over 3–4 months, with written tests to gauge the information flow. The average patient will find the latter a bit much and may become so intimidated by the formality that they decide pump therapy is just not for them. A combination of individual and group sessions may work well because many patients benefit from group interaction. Success begets success, and clinicians are likely to design and implement what they have found works best for their patients.

A group class covering some of the pump education topics can also be time-efficient for the healthcare professional/team. Ideally, patients should have sessions with an endocrinologist and a CDE, who can be a registered dietitian (RD), registered nurse (RN), registered pharmacist (RPh), or exercise physiologist, and has experience with pump therapy. Consultation with a psychologist, who specializes in diabetes and understands pump therapy is also extremely useful.

Another consideration for pump readiness is to recommend that your potential pump patient attend a local pump support group. Most pump support groups are facilitated by a pump-savvy CDE who can manage the tone of the overall group and keep the focus on the topic(s) being discussed. The caveat to attending a pump support group is that, depending on the patients who are present, potential pump patients may become inappropriately excited hearing how "easy" pump therapy is. On the other hand, potential patients may become so dismayed by complaints that they decide pump therapy isn't for them. In both cases, pump therapy reality lies somewhere between the supportive successful pump patient and the unhappy struggling pump patient. Many clinicians recommend potential pumpers attend at least two support group meetings before making the final decision to choose pump therapy.

There are education components that will guarantee successful pump therapy. Although the patient's education begins as you present the "Steps for Helping the Patient Determine and Achieve Readiness" (Chapter 3), once a decision to proceed with pump therapy occurs, new educational objectives emerge:

- Establishing goals
- Learning carbohydrate counting (if this is new to the patient)
- Calculating insulin-to-carbohydrate ratio(s) (ICR) (if this is new to the patient)
- Calculating the correction (sensitivity) factor(s) (CF) (if this is new to the patient)
- Managing hyperglycemia and hypoglycemia
- Choosing and inserting infusion sets
- Coping with lifestyle issues, sick days, exercise, supplies, and travel

A patient reference published by the American Diabetes Association, *Insulin Pumps and Continuous Glucose Monitoring* (Kaufman 2012) can be of great assistance to your patients as they learn the details of pump therapy.

Review or establish appropriate blood glucose and A1C targets with the patient at this time (Tables 2 and 3) (ADA 2013). Emphasize that pump therapy does not guarantee an automatic improvement in control but may make achieving control easier while providing a more flexible lifestyle. The responsibility for the improvements patients make using this new tool rests in their hands. Patients who are not doing well on MDI therapy may embrace the greater lifestyle flexibility offered by insulin pump therapy and become willing to put forth the effort needed for success.

Discuss how critical it is for the patient to keep detailed records during the prepump education and pump start-up periods, which could last 1–4 months or longer. SMBG should include frequent pre- and postprandial blood glucose checks, at least four times a day, including one middle-of-the-night check around 3:00 a.m.

| TABLE 2. Glycemic Recommendations for Nonpregnant Adults with Diabetes* | |
|---|---|
| Preprandial capillary plasma glucose (mg/dl) | 70–130* |
| Peak postprandial capillary plasma glucose (mg/dl) | <180* |
| A1C (%) | <7* |
| Goals should be individualized based on: | |
|     duration of diabetes | |
|     age/life expectancy | |
|     comorbid conditions | |
|     known CVD or advanced microvascular complications | |
|     hypoglycemia unawareness | |
|     individual patient considerations | |

*More- or less-stringent glycemic goals may be appropriate for individual patients.
Postprandial glucose may be targeted if A1C goals are not met despite teaching preprandial glucose goals.
Postprandial glucose measurements should be made 1–2 h after the beginning of the meal, generally peak levels in patients with diabetes.

## TABLE 3. Plasma Blood Glucose and A1C Goals for Type 1 Diabetes by Age Group*

| (ADA 2013) | Plasma Blood Glucose Goal Range (mg/dl) | | | |
|---|---|---|---|---|
| Values by age (years) | Before Meals | Bedtime/ Overnight | A1C | Rationale |
| Toddlers and Preschoolers (0–6) | 100–180 | 110–200 | <8.5% | Vulnerability to hypoglycemia, insulin sensitivity, unpredictability in dietary intake and physical activity; a lower goal (<8.0%) is reasonable if it can be achieved without excessive hypoglycemia |
| School age (6–12) | 90–180 | 90–150 | <8.0% | Vulnerability to hypoglycemia; a lower goal (<7.5%) is reasonable if it can be achieved without excessive hypoglycemia |
| Adolescents and young adults (13–19) | 90–130 | 90–150 | <7.5% | A lower goal (<7.0%) is reasonable if it can be achieved without excessive hypoglycemia |

*In setting glycemic goals for children:
Goals should be individualized and lower goals may be reasonable based on benefit risk assessment.
Blood glucose goals should be modified in children with frequent hypoglycemia or hypoglycemia unawareness.
Postprandial blood glucose values should be measured when there is a discrepancy between preprandial blood glucose values and A1C levels and to help assess glycemia in those on basal/bolus regimens.

For enhanced pattern recognition purposes, ask the patient to also record factors that affect blood glucose, such as:

- Dietary intake, including grams of carbohydrate at each meal and snack
- Insulin doses (basal rates and bolus doses)
- Exercise: intensity, duration, and time of day
- Stress

■ Illness

■ Menstrual cycle

Patients who are already performing active self-management with MDI make the transition to pump therapy fairly easily. The challenges lie in what is common to both MDI and pump therapy—learning carb counting, planning ahead, adjusting doses for lifestyle issues, etc.

## Patients Who Are Using Continuous Glucose Monitoring

CGM is another tool that may be helpful to you in determining your patient's pattern of blood glucose control and deciding on initial pump basal rate(s) and bolus doses. Keep in mind the CGM measures glucose in interstitial fluid, not blood, so the values obtained at the same time from CGM and SMBG may not be identical. Refer to Chapter 6 for more on CGM.

Remind the patient of the learning curve associated with something as new and detailed as pump therapy initiation. Today's "smart pumps" allow for easier determination of appropriate bolus doses and decision-making associated with pump therapy, but even the smartest of pumps cannot replace knowledge of the "hows" and "whys" of diabetes education and management. Make assurances that with time and experience, the patient will earn the freedom of being able to interpret his or her results and make safe self-management decisions using their insulin pump.

# Carbohydrate Counting

**It is essential that the patient, or parents if the patient is a child, learn and use advanced carbohydrate counting skills for several weeks or months before beginning pump therapy.** It is both the prescribing clinician's responsibility as well as the potential pump user's responsibility that the prospective pumper has proficiency in advanced carbohydrate counting. Mastery of advanced carbohydrate counting skills requires instruction from an RD, preferably a CDE with pump therapy experience, and usually takes a few weeks to learn, depending on the patient's history and abilities.

A person's knowledge of carbohydrate counting and their comfort level with adjusting prandial (bolus insulin doses) will provide a foundation for success with insulin pump therapy. Many HCPs and prospective pumpers alike do not realize that this is the responsibility of the pump prescriber and pumper/parents. Teaching advanced carbohydrate counting skills is not the responsibility of a contracted per diem pump trainer or pump manufacturer employee (sales representative, territory manager, clinical education specialist, clinical manager, etc.) on the day of the pump therapy training or initiation. At this point, it is too late in the process to begin teaching carbohydrate-counting methods and concepts. Ideally, a prospective pumper should be able to demonstrate advanced carbohydrate-counting skills weeks or months BEFORE beginning pump therapy.

After initial review with the prospective pumper/parents, use follow-up session(s) as necessary to validate the patient's/parents' ability to count carbohydrate grams accurately. For additional information, refer to the American Diabetes Association book *Practical Carbohydrate Counting: A How-to-Teach Guide for Health Professionals* (Warshaw 2008). Although some pumps offer a carbohydrate gram database of commonly eaten foods, every pump patient should know how to accurately count carbohydrate grams of their favorite foods and be able to manually calculate a bolus insulin dose based on their specific insulin-to-carbohydrate ratio(s). Smartphones and thinkpads allow the downloading of a variety of useful carbohydrate applications that serve as a reference source for unfamiliar foods or restaurant meals. Some pumps offer the ability for the user to build a personalized food database of commonly eaten favorite foods and beverages and then program these as preset amounts with user-assigned names, such as "pancake breakfast" or "dinner salad."

Another innovative pump option allows the user to simply input the meal items to be consumed; the pump adds the carbohydrate grams, and based on personalized information programmed by the user, calculates the appropriate carbohydrate bolus. Regardless of the manner in which a pump user totals his/her meal and snack carbohydrate amounts, it is essential that the user understand how to use an insulin-to-carbohydrate ratio(s).

Food labels provide the total carbohydrate grams, but if the patient is not accurate in knowing the carb amounts of the portions s/he is eating (i.e., adding up the total grams of carbohydrate in their meal or snack), the bolus insulin dose will not be correct. Stress the importance of **accurate measurements** and knowing how to use insulin-to-carbohydrate ratio(s) consistently.

**Is the Patient Ready?**

A prospective pump candidate should be adept at answering the following questions related to carbohydrate counting and insulin pump therapy without hesitation:

1. Do you know which foods contain carbohydrate?
2. How do you know how much carbohydrate you eat? (i.e., how do you count carbohydrate?)
3. How do you determine your premeal insulin doses?
4. What is (are) your insulin-to-carbohydrate ratio(s)?
5. Do you know how long your insulin (dose[s]) lasts?
6. How do you treat your high blood glucose levels?
7. What is (are) your correction (or insulin sensitivity) factor(s)?
8. How do you treat hypoglycemia?

There are countless stories of "pump therapy failures" or people whose pump therapy "just didn't work right," etc. Many of these disheartening tales of failed pump therapy can easily be traced to lack of carbohydrate-counting skills coupled with inaccurate basal doses, or, worse yet, one constant hourly basal rate for 24 hours. There are even cases of people using an insulin pump with a set bolus dose per meal (often referred to as "a very expensive insulin pen or syringe") without any regard to the amount of carbohydrate to be consumed. Again, **it is essential that the patient or parents if the patient is a child, master carbohydrate counting before beginning pump therapy. It is a must for successful pump therapy.**

For specifics on calculating insulin-to-carbohydrate ratios, see Calculating Insulin-to-Carbohydrate Ratios in Chapter 5.

# Hyperglycemia

Remind the patient that the pump uses only rapid-acting insulin, and if there is an unexpected or accidental interruption of basal insulin delivery or an inaccurate or missed bolus, hyperglycemia can occur. Other causes of hyperglycemia during pump therapy include infusion set issues, such as cracked or broken tubing or tubing that has become disconnected from the pump or infusion site; or leaving the infusion set in (or pod on) too long. Expired insulin, or insulin in the pump cartridge/reservoir that has been exposed to heat and become less effective, can lead to elevated blood glucose levels. Ignoring warnings or alerts for a low or dead battery, illness, stress, onset of menses, and a change in pump settings with time zone changes can also cause hyperglycemia.

You will be surprised (disheartened) at how many patients with type 1 diabetes are not familiar with ketones (cause, treatment, and prevention) and the use of ketone test strips. Educate your patients on the importance of obtaining ketone test strips, when to use them, and to make sure they periodically check their expiration date. Although ketone test strips are available over-the-counter, your patient may request or require a prescription for insurance reimbursement. Blood ketone strips require a meter. Now is a good time to provide a (new) prescription for a vial or pen of long-acting insulin. Also, make sure the patient has rapid-acting insulin readily available in case of infusion site or pump issues/malfunctions. Stress the importance of carrying a spare infusion set or pod. Many people find it upsetting to know they need to always carry their "emergency" or back-up "kit," but the first time a pump patient experiences severe hyperglycemia during pump therapy, they quickly appreciate the importance of being prepared.

# Hypoglycemia

Education on hypoglycemia management includes a review of the causes, prevention, and treatment. A review of symptoms at this time is also helpful. Remind the patient that the insulin pump does not "think" and cannot prevent hypoglycemia. A miscalculated bolus dose (which can also be a result of inaccurate carb counting), "stacking insulin" (see Chapter 5), inaccurate basal rates, changes in pump settings due to time zone changes, and planned or unplanned exercise can cause hypoglycemia.

For mild to moderate hypoglycemia, teach and emphasize the Rule of 15:

- Treat hypoglycemia with 15 g fast-acting carbohydrate
- Check blood glucose after 15 minutes
- Repeat the treatment as needed

**Every insulin-using patient should have a glucagon prescription.** Instructions on its use should be provided to the patient's family members, friends, and/or significant other(s) (including coworkers). This information should not be new to the patient or to the people around him or her.

Additionally, now is also a good time to review the importance of wearing easily visible **medical identification.** There are many choices, including inexpensive necklaces, bracelets, charms, and pendants for both women and men, as well as the option of more expensive and/or custom-made engraved medical jewelry. Again, this should not be new to the patient, but is often an overlooked yet very important factor in living with diabetes.

# Infusion Set Insertion

The patient may have already observed the insertion and removal of an infusion set when deciding whether or not to try pump therapy (see Chapter 3, Pump Candidate Basics). If not, the patient should see a demonstration, and may benefit from a practice insertion, especially if s/he is anxious about inserting or wearing an infusion set. During pump start-up, the patient will learn how to prepare the skin and insert the infusion set. Pump manufacturer personnel also provide specific instructions and detailed information to pump patients about infusion set insertion procedures.

The abdomen is the preferred infusion site because it offers a consistent rate of absorption. However, pump patients have had success using other subcutaneous sites, e.g., the upper hip/buttock, thigh, and upper arm. Teach patients to avoid inserting the set within a 2-inch diameter of the navel, at the waistline or belt area, or in any area where clothing would rub against or constrict the site.

Infusion sets must be changed every 1–3 days (1–2 days for metal/steel and 2–3 days for Teflon or soft cannula) to prevent infection and scar tissue buildup, which can lead to occlusions and reduce or interrupt delivery of insulin. The site should be rotated every time the infusion set base or pod is replaced, usually from one side of the body to the other, and ½ to 1 inch away from a previous site. The patient must check the site at least once daily for redness, tenderness, and tape or dressing placement. Encourage patients with long-term diabetes, or those with possible long-term use and resultant scar tissue of their abdominal area from injections, to consider alternative subcutaneous infusion sites. Alternative sites include the upper arm, upper thigh, and upper buttocal area. Patients who have been using CGM also may have favorite injection sites and will have limited choices for pump infusion site placement. It is important to emphasize site rotation and adherence to frequent (2–3 day) site changes. You should check a patient's infusion sites at every visit to be sure the patient is not developing lipohypertrophy, which often results from inadequate site rotation.

## Patch/Pod Pump Infusion Set

Presently, a patch pump infusion set is of the soft cannula type and would be inserted similarly to an infusion set base that has connecting tubing. The self-adhesive tape for a pod pump has stronger adhesive to prevent dislodgement during activities or water exposure. Newer "modular type" models on the horizon may require only the infusion catheter to be replaced, allowing the pump pod to be reused and thus, reducing the expense of replacing the entire pod.

## Steps for Infusion Set Insertion

1. Wash hands with antibacterial soap.
2. Assemble the infusion set supplies in a well-lit, clean workspace.
3. Prepare the infusion site using an antibacterial soap or solution or a commercial product, such as an IV Prep pad, Betadine pad, Betadine solution (iodine), or Hibiclens (chlorhexiden). Allow the skin to dry naturally. Anxious children and apprehensive adults may benefit from the use of a topical analgesic (including ice, a cold spoon, or a cold beverage can/bottle) to numb the skin before inserting the infusion set. Products to reduce discomfort from the infusion set base or pod insertion include over-the-counter creams, such as LMX4 and Numby Stuff, and a prescription cream called EMLA. Pump manufacturers can provide a list of commonly used skin prep products.
4. Follow the manufacturer's instructions for the infusion set insertion and needle removal (if using a Teflon cannula set).
5. Secure the set/pod to the site with the sterile self-adhesive tape/dressing.
6. Follow the manufacturer's instructions to attach the tubing and bolus insulin to fill the cannula.

A metal/steel needle set may be felt, whereas a Teflon cannula set will not. If a set becomes uncomfortable after it is in position, it should be removed and discarded, and a new one should be inserted in a different site. If the site becomes red, swollen, irritated, or painful, the patient should remove and discard the set and rotate the site. The set should also be changed if blood appears in the tubing.

## Optional Saline Trial

An optional saline trial can be done with a loaner (or demo model) pump while patients are deciding whether a pump is the right tool for them or after the pump is purchased and delivered during the pump preparation period. A saline trial may help the patient decide which pump to choose (see Chapter 2). People who are unsure about "being attached to something 24 h a day" or have anxiety about infusion set insertion may find that wearing a pump with saline allays fears and concerns. A saline trial also provides the patient the opportunity to learn the functions of the pump (the "buttonology") without feeling the pressure of "If I press this button, I might make a mistake." The insulin start that follows a saline trial may serve as a review of the technical training of the pump initiation process. This may be beneficial to those patients who are not quick learners or who express nervousness or anxiety about their actual pump start.

A saline trial should not be mandatory. MDI therapy must continue while wearing a saline pump; therefore, the patient does twice the work without enjoying the flexibility or freedom associated with pump therapy. And a patient who is excited about pump therapy is impatient to get started. A pump patient who is required by his or her clinician or CDE to wear the pump with saline first may resent the delay in the pump start and view it as a waste of time. The clinician and patient, or parents of the pediatric patient, should decide together if a saline start is truly appropriate. Saline requires a prescription, which the prescribing physician must provide to the patient.

## Lifestyle Issues and Wearing the Pump

Many prospective pump users hesitate or neglect to ask about lifestyle concerns; therefore, the healthcare professional must take the initiative and include this information in the pump education process.

## Daily Wear

The pump can be worn by several different means, including a clip, a case (leather, vinyl, or plastic) with or without a built-in clip or belt loops, or inside clothing such as thigh or leg garments, boxer shorts, lounging pants, and slips with pump pouches or pockets. A cotton infant sock is another option: the pump fits into the sock easily and can be worn in the side or cup of a bra, under control-top pantyhose or other shapewear-type undergarments, or pinned inside clothing. Some patients wear the pump in the top of their foot sock with long infusion set tubing under their slacks/trousers and use a remote feature or cross their legs and use the touch bolus button to deliver bolus insulin as needed. Another option is to sew pockets into the seams of garments or use Velcro for removable pockets. There are companies that manufacture devices that even roll up the pump tubing (refer to Chapter 8, Forms and Resources). Ask the pump patient in training to think ahead about wearing the pump with various types of clothing and in different situations, such as getting dressed and using the bathroom (toilet). An insulin pump pod, or "tubeless" pump is attached directly to the skin and does not require use of a case or clip.

## Sleeping

Every prospective pump user wonders what to do with the pump during sleep. The patient may want to try wearing the pump inside the pocket of pajamas, a nightshirt, a nightgown, or boxer shorts. Another option, depending on the length of the tubing, is placing the pump in a specific location, such as under the pillow or on a night table. The pump can also be clipped to a sheet or blanket or placed freely in the bed. Longer tubing provides greater flexibility for moving and turning. Reassure the pump patient that even if the tubing is knotted upon awakening, insulin delivery will not be disturbed. The infusion set/pod dressing or tape secures the infusion set safely to the site.

Use of an electric blanket can affect the potency of insulin, especially if the pump is directly on the heating coils. Pump users need to consider this if their fasting blood glucose is erratic without explanation.

## Bathing/Showering

Pumps are waterproof or water resistant—check with the pump manufacturer for specific guidelines. Even if the pump patient is not planning on wearing the pump while bathing or showering, pumps have been known to fall in the toilet.

With a disconnect infusion set, the pump can be disconnected for up to 1 h and reconnected after bathing or showering. Remind the patient that insulin is very heat sensitive; soaking in a hot bath or whirlpool or using a sauna while wearing the pump is not recommended.

## Intimacy/Sexual Activity

To wear the pump or not during sexual activity is the patient's choice. If the patient wants to keep the pump connected, longer infusion set tubing may be recommended or preferred. The patient should be reminded to reconnect his or her infusion set and pump and the infusion site should always be checked to make certain the set base has remained intact. See "Intimacy/Sexual Activity" on page 129 for additional information.

## Sports/Physical Exercise

Advise the patient that an insulin pump can, and should be worn during exercise and physical activity, and even professional athletes keep their pumps attached while engaged in their sport of choice. Specific suggestions for wearing the pump and guidelines for adjusting insulin doses during exercise are provided in "Exercise and Physical Activity" on page 122.

## Medical Procedures, Sick Days/Illness, and Hospitalization

The specific medical procedure (CAT scan, X-ray, etc.) will determine whether or not the pump should be worn. Patients may also be advised prior to the medical procedure or test if it is appropriate for the pump to be exposed to the medical test or procedure. Remind the patient that if the pump is to be disconnected longer than an hour, it may be necessary to make adjustments in insulin doses.

Advise patients that, similar to MDI therapy, lengthy medical procedures and sick days and illness often require adjustments in insulin doses and the same guidelines will apply. A prospective pump patient may ask if they can wear their pump while ill—reassure the patient that illness does not require the pump to be disconnected, but in the case of severe illness or if the patient is incapable of operating their pump, s/he may require the assistance of another person and/or a temporary return to MDI therapy. A back-up, or "pre-pump" plan is essential.

Refer to "Managing Sick Days and Medical Procedures" on page 130 , for specifics on managing pump therapy during medical procedures, sick days, and hospitalization.

# Patient Support System

Pump therapy initiation can be an emotional process for the patient. It may have taken a patient several months or even years to make the decision to choose pump therapy. In addition to your support and encouragement, the patient's personal support system is an important factor in successful pump therapy. Spouse/significant other and family encouragement will help the patient in his/her pump education and initiation process. The patient may choose to also involve friends and co-workers, and may invite them to co-attend pump support group meetings, or at the least, may inform them of this life-changing decision. Diabetes-focused consumer magazines and publications are other materials the patient may find helpful. Social media are another avenue of support, and the availability of information on the internet is astounding. There are many internet resources related to insulin pump therapy, and patients may find or be directed to various insulin pump sites and blogs. You can also provide reliable credible resources (see Chapter 8, Forms and Resources). Pump manufacturers offer support via internet, print, and telephone and can serve as a great resource to a new pump patient.

# Ordering the Pump and Supplies

Once you and the patient have decided to initiate pump therapy and the patient is close to "being ready" (refer to preceding chapters), the next step is to order the pump and supplies. Insurance companies and pump manufacturers vary in the pump order process. Pump companies have designated personnel who walk the patient through the order process. Depending on the company's policies and procedures, as well as those of the patient's insurance company, the process can take anywhere from a few days to a few weeks. A signed order or prescription for the pump and initial supplies (infusion sets or pods, cartridges/reservoirs, tape, skin prep) from the healthcare professional is required, and additional paperwork may be requested. This may include, but is not limited to: a letter of medical necessity, usually with "check-off boxes" related to the patient's diabetes control status and/or complications; SMBG data maintained by the patient or available from you; and recent and past A1C results. Additionally, the pump order may also include instructions for the pump start and initial settings, including blood glucose targets, basal rate(s), insulin-to-carb ratio(s), correction factor(s), and duration of insulin action ("insulin on board"). A prescription for saline is required if a saline pump start is desirable, and a prescription for rapid-acting insulin, taking into account the additional amount needed for tubing, is a must.

A logistic consideration is the designation of the pump delivery. Some clinicians prefer the pump be delivered to them rather than to the patient, as some patients have self-initiated without the knowledge of their prescribing physician and without any training, with disastrous results. In this case, the healthcare professional is responsible for informing the patient that the pump has been delivered and training by the pump manufacturer (CDE trainer) can be scheduled. Another "order" is to designate who will "follow" the patient, i.e., adjust insulin doses during pump initiation, usually the first few weeks. You must decide if you will be in frequent communication with the patient during the initiation period, or if you prefer the pump company to manage this. Pump manufacturers may offer initial follow-up as a service provided by their staff or per diem CDE.

## Pump Supplies

The initial pump order includes not only the insulin pump, but also the supplies necessary for the patient to get started. These include cartridges/reservoirs; infusion sets or pods; dressing/tape, such as IV 3000, skin prep, such as IV Prep, and battery. An initial pump order also includes user guide instructions, such as online tools, DVDs, and printed booklets.

Most pump orders request a 3-month supply, so keep this in mind when completing the initial pump order or prescription. Consider that the cartridges/reservoirs and infusion set/pods will be changed every 1 to 3 days, so do the math. On the average, an infusion set is changed every 2 to 3 days; in one month, the pump user may need 10 to 15 cartridges/reservoirs and infusion sets/pods, and a 3-month supply may be a standard order. There may be more set and site changes initially as the new pump user may "lose" some sets during their learning curve. The same is true for the insulin. Remember that the tubing contains insulin, so when the patient changes their infusion set tubing, the insulin in the tubing is also discarded. One inch of tubing contains 0.3 to 0.5 units of insulin (depending on the brand of infusion set), so discarding 43″ tubing every 2 days results in a loss of over 250 units of insulin per month. Over time, some patients have learned to change only the actual infusion set base, leaving the tubing attached to their cartridge/reservoir until the cartridge is depleted. As of this publication date, the rapid-acting insulin analogs are FDA-approved for use in an insulin pump cartridge/reservoir for several days, including: Apidra®, 48 hours; Humalog®, up to seven days (three in the tubing); and NovoLog®, up to six days (sanofi-aventis 2009; Eli Lilly 2011; Novo Nordisk 2002–2011). But a decrease in efficacy, resulting in escalating hyperglycemia, can occur if the insulin remains in the cartridge/reservoir too long; cautionary advice is recommended. During initial pump starts, recommend patients "change everything" every 2 to 3 days. This will help patients to learn proper procedures and improve their technique, and will also eliminate the possibility of ineffective insulin as a cause of hyperglycemia. Refer to "Infusion Site and Tubing Concerns" in Chapter 6 for additional information.

## REFERENCES

American Diabetes Association: 2013 Clinical practice recommendations. *Diabetes Care* 36:S11–S66, 2013

Eli Lilly and Company: *Humalog (insulin lispro injection USP [rDNA origin]) for Injection Prescribing Information.* Indianapolis, IN: Eli Lilly and Company, 2011

Kaufman FR, Westfall E: *Insulin Pumps and Continuous Glucose Monitoring: A User's Guide to Effective Diabetes Management,* Alexandria VA: American Diabetes Association, 2012

Novo Nordisk A/S: *NovoLog® (insulin aspart [rDNA origin]) Injection Prescribing Information.* Novo Nordisk A/S, Bagsvaerd, Denmark, 2002–2011

Roche Insulin Delivery Systems, Inc.: *ACCU-CHEK Guide to Infusion Site Management.* Fishers,IN: 2012

sanofi-aventis: *Apidra (insulin gluslisine [rDNA origin] injection) solution for injection Prescribing Information.* Bridgewater, NJ: sanofi-aventis U.S., 2009

## CHAPTER 5

# Pump Start-Up

NICHOLAS B. ARGENTO, MD
KAREN M. BOLDERMAN, RD, LDN, CDE

## Pump Start Basics: Patient and Prescriber Responsibilities

The first questions for you to answer are:

1. who is going to be responsible for the initial pump training?;
2. who is going to provide first-line support in helping the patient make the initial transition from injections to the pump, including making the initial pump adjustments?

Increasingly, pump companies may both provide services to the new pump patient and take responsibility for the transition, training, and initial pump adjustments with physician authorization, which may be a good idea for small offices or centers that do not have the personnel who can provide these services. Some pump companies employ clinicians, i.e., HCPs (RD, RN, or RPh) who are usually CDEs for this role, while others use consultant CDEs to train and/or manage insulin pump patients. If you opt to have a third party provide the training and early followup, it would be important to meet with representatives of the third party to make sure there is a clear understanding by both parties of who is providing specific services, how followup will be provided, what kind of progress reports you can expect, a procedure for dealing with emergencies, and when the third party would stop providing initial guidance and turn the responsibility for routine followup back to you. Check with your local pump sales representatives and/or clinicians on availability if they would like to assume this responsibility.

Typically, the pump start-up education session takes 2–4 h and requires the undivided attention of the pump user or parent(s). Pump training should nearly always be done in an outpatient setting, such as the clinician's office or the patient's home, with permission and approval of the prescribing physician (if the pump company personnel performing the training offers home training as an option). Because of concerns about security issues with home training, it may not be the best option, or even available, in some areas. Inpatient admissions should rarely be necessary unless adequate support and monitoring are not available in the home setting. An inpatient admission is usually for one overnight stay, allowing close monitoring of nocturnal and fasting blood glucose levels, and may be most beneficial for children or pregnant women with unstable glycemic control. Another option is the "23-h observational stay," i.e., the patient is trained, monitored, and discharged 1 h short of a 24-h stay, thus avoiding charges for and a record of a hospital admission. The patient should verify his/her insurance coverage, as insurance pre-approval may be required for any inpatient pump training.

Carefully set the pump start-up date. Make sure that the patient's first few weeks of pump therapy are planned for a time when they are likely to be in a normal routine. The patient should avoid situations or conditions that may adversely affect blood glucose levels or interfere with the establishment of basal rates, such as:

- Pre-menses or menstruation
- Out-of-town or unusual travel
- Unusual work, school, or leisure-activity schedules
- Moderate-to-strenuous exercise, including major sports activities
- Outpatient surgery, including dental work
- Holidays
- Limited access to telephone and/or email/fax communication

Pump start-up orders must be provided to the patient several days in advance. Most endocrinologists and CDEs use forms to provide instructions for "weaning" the patient off intermediate- or long-acting insulin. Other written instructions for the patient include self-monitoring blood glucose and dietary guidelines, a list of supplies to bring to the pump start-up appointment, and specific information regarding appointment time and location (see Chapter 8, Forms and Resources).

Because the pump start is best initiated without the interference of any lasting effect of intermediate- or long-acting insulin, the start is usually scheduled in the morning after the patient has taken his or her rapid- or fast-acting insulin to cover the breakfast meal. The last dose of intermediate insulin (NPH) should be administered at least 12 h before the scheduled pump start. The bedtime dose can be given as usual the evening before the pump start because the actual "hook up" to the pump occurs at the end of the start-up training period late the next morning. The patient should administer the last dose of long-acting insulin (insulin glargine or insulin detemir) 24 h in advance, if possible. Since there may be some basal insulin effect still present on the start day, the basal rate can be reduced for the first 6–12 hours by 30%. Some clinicians choose to continue the long-acting insulin and decrease the dose by 50% the day preceding the pump start, though this will lead to higher than normal blood glucose levels the morning prior to pump start. Another option is to discontinue the insulin glargine or insulin detemir 36 h in advance of the pump start, substituting a calculated dose of NPH insulin the night before the pump start. It is not advisable to discontinue intermediate- or long-acting insulin and substitute with multiple doses of rapid-acting insulin every 3–4 h throughout the night before the pump start. The result will be a tired and "out-of-sorts" patient whose sleep has been disrupted.

# Pump Start Guidelines for the Patient

On the pump start day, the patient should:

1. Eat a usual breakfast, following appropriate rapid- or short-acting insulin injection.
2. Wear comfortable two-piece clothing, not dresses or one-piece garments.
3. Bring the following items:
   - New vial of prescribed rapid-acting insulin analog at room temperature. A partially used vial should not be used unless it was recently opened

and there is no chance it was mixed/contaminated inadvertently with an intermediate or long-acting insulin.

- Glucose meter, lancets, lancet device, glucose test strips
- Glucose log book or SMBG records
- Hypoglycemia treatment
- Calculator
- Paper and pen
- Target glycemic levels, insulin-to-carbohydrate ratio (ICR), correction or (insulin sensitivity) factor [CF] duration of insulin action, and SMBG instructions (as agreed upon by prescriber and patient)

4. Come ready for a several-hour education session.

If the patient received the pump at home, s/he should check the contents of the box with shipping information several days in advance of the pump start. Emphasize to the patient that s/he needs to bring the entire box with all contents and supplies to the pump start. Each pump shipment should contain:

- New pump and, if appropriate, remote device or pod controller/PDM
- Batteries
- Pump cartridges/reservoirs or pods
- Skin prep product(s)
- Infusion sets or pods
- Infusion set inserter device, if appropriate
- Infusion site dressings, if appropriate
- User's manual
- Instructional DVD or CD if available
- Warranty card/information
- Additional written materials (e.g., accessory catalogs, special instructions)

# Pump Start Guidelines for the Clinician

If the pump and corresponding supplies were shipped to the clinician's site, open the box and inspect it for completeness (as outlined above) several days preceding the pump start.

An insulin pump start-up training session includes a review of the pump, accessories, and instructions for use:

- Inserting and removing the batteries
- Filling (if appropriate) and placing the pump insulin cartridge/reservoir or pod
- Attaching the infusion set tubing to the pump, if applicable
- Priming the tubing or pod, i.e., filling the infusion set tubing or pod with insulin
- Programming the pump ("buttonology" training) and setting all applicable features (as available per pump model), such as clock, date, sound volume, language, alarm type, screen light; basal rates with limits and temporary basal type; bolus increments, bolus delivery duration, bolus calculator settings with targets; insulin-to-carbohydrate ratio(s) [ICR], correction/insulin sensitivity factor(s) [CF/ISF], insulin "on board"/duration of insulin action; pump suspension/stop, memory/history, reviewing waterproof specifics; and any other settings applicable to that particular pump.
- Delivering a bolus into midair for practice
- Stopping a bolus mid-delivery
- Recognizing and acting on any warnings or alarms
- Preparing the infusion site
- Inserting the infusion set (using insertion device, if applicable) or pod
- Inspecting the infusion set
- Discussing the troubleshooting guidelines, i.e., reviewing technical problems that can occur with the pump and/or infusion site and set or pod, such as site tenderness, loose tape, tubing leakage, or air bubbles in tubing, if applicable
- Reviewing the user's manual and completing the pump warranty information
- Reviewing of any other accompanying pump manufacturer literature, including accessory catalogs, specific instructions, or technical changes that do not appear in the user's manual
- Identifying the contact names and numbers of pump manufacturer representatives or customer service for technical assistance (see Chapter 8, Forms and Resources)

- Reviewing follow-up and management guidelines as outlined by the prescribing physician, including target glycemic levels, insulin-to-carbohydrate ratio(s), correction factor(s), and contact names and numbers (see Chapter 8, Forms and Resources)
- Completing pump training checklist with copies to other healthcare team members as appropriate

The clinician is responsible for providing or signing off on pump start orders to the diabetes educator or designated pump trainer providing the pump start-up training. These include:

- Starting basal rate(s)
- Insulin-to-carbohydrate ratio(s)
- Correction (or sensitivity) factor(s) and instructions for use (may delay implementation until basal rates have been fine-tuned)
- Duration of insulin action ("insulin on board" duration)
- SMBG instructions
- Communication guidelines, i.e., who, when, and where the patient contacts for reporting SMBG results/asking for diabetes management assistance (HCPs) and asking for technical assistance (pump manufacturer)

# Determining Target Blood Glucose Values

Target preprandial blood glucose levels for nonpregnant adults are between 70–130 mg/dl, and a peak 1–2 h postprandial blood glucose below 180 mg/dl (American Diabetes Association 2013). The American Association of Clinical Endocrinologists (AACE) uses the more aggressive goals of pre-prandial blood glucose levels below 110 mg/dl, and 1 h postprandial blood glucose below 140 mg/dl (Handelsman 2011). Both the ADA and AACE acknowledge the importance of goal individualization by noting that higher goals may be appropriate for patients who are prone to hypoglycemia, have hypoglycemic unawareness, have a high burden of comorbidities, or have a limited life span. Lower goals are necessary for women who are contemplating pregnancy or are pregnant (Kitzmiller 2008; ADA 2013).

It is important that you specify glycemic goals for the patient. Smart pumps allow a target blood glucose value or range to be entered, which is really a preprandial target. The specifics of how the different pump systems use the target value to calculate a recommended dose of insulin vary, and some of the specific features can be individualized to some extent with each pump. It is important to understand the specifics of the system your patient will be using. For example, a pump may allow a single target value, e.g., 110 mg/dl, or a single target value but only add or subtract insulin if the value is outside of a specified range that is set around that value, e.g., 110 +/− 15 mg/dl, so the range would be 95 to 125 mg/dl, but the calculation would correct to 110 mg/dl in its dosing recommendations if the current value entered is outside of that range. Another system might allow a range, for example 100–120 mg/dl, and calculate an insulin dose to reach the range, but not the midpoint of the range. Yet, another pump system may use the midpoint of an entered range as the blood glucose target.

## Example 1: Blood Glucose Target

ICR: 1 unit to 10 g; CF: 40 mg/dl; target blood glucose: 100 mg/dl with no range set
Preprandial blood glucose 150 mg/dl, consuming 45 g carbohydrate, no "insulin on board"

*Recommended dose:*
45 g ÷ 10 = 4.5 units for carbohydrate, plus
150 mg/dl − 100 mg/dl = 50 mg/dl above target range ÷ CF = 50 ÷ 40 = 1.25 units, so 1.25 units for correction of hyperglycemia, thus
Insulin to cover carbohydrate + correction insulin = 4.5 units + 1.25 units = 5.75 units as the recommended total bolus

## Example 2: Blood Glucose Target Range

ICR: 1 unit to 10 g; CF: 40 mg/dl; target blood glucose range: 90–110 mg/dl
Preprandial blood glucose 150 mg/dl, consuming 45 g carbohydrate, no "insulin on board."

*Recommended dose:*
45 g ÷ 10 = 4.5 units for carbohydrate, plus
150 mg/dl − 110 mg/dl = 40 mg/dl above target range, 40 ÷ 40 = 1.0 unit for correction of hyperglycemia, thus

Insulin to cover carbohydrate + correction insulin = 4.5 units
+ 1.0 units = 5.5 units as the recommended total bolus

## Example 3: Blood Glucose Target Range

ICR: 1 unit to 10 g; CF: 40 mg/dl; target blood glucose: 100 mg/dl with range set as +/− 15 mg/dl
Pre-prandial blood glucose 150 mg/dl, consuming 45 g carbohydrate, no "insulin on board."

*Recommended dose:*

45 g ÷ 10 = 4.5 units for carbohydrate, plus
150 mg/dl − 100 mg/dl = 50 mg/dl above target ÷ CF = 50 ÷ 40 =
1.25, so 1.25 units for correction of hyperglycemia, thus
Insulin to cover carbohydrate + correction insulin= 4.5 units + 1.25
units = 5.75 units as the recommended total bolus

## Example 4: Blood Glucose Target Range

ICR: 1 unit to 10 g; CF: 40; target blood glucose: 100 mg/dl with range set as +/− 15 mg/dl
Preprandial blood glucose 114 mg/dl, eating 45 g carbohydrate, no "insulin on board."

*Recommended dose:*

45 g ÷ 10 = 4.5 units for carbohydrate, plus
114 mg/dl − 100 mg/dl = 14 mg/dl above target, but since the blood
glucose is within the target range specified, no correction dose
recommended; thus
Insulin to cover carbohydrate + correction insulin = 4.5 units + 0 units
= 4.5 units as the total recommended bolus

Many clinicians use a blood glucose goal for nonpregnant adults of 100 mg/dl or 90–110 mg/dl, but a higher goal, such as 120–130 mg/dl, may be set if the patient is new to pump therapy or has had recurrent hypoglycemia. Smart pumps also allow setting different target glucose values for different times of the day, which is a useful feature that allows setting a higher target before bedtime, in order to reduce the risk of nocturnal hypoglycemia.

# Determining Starting Basal Rate

The basal rate is usually 40–50% of the total daily dose (TDD), with the remainder comprised of bolus insulin doses. It is important to verify that the patient was actually adhering to the prescribed doses when determining a TDD, because the actual TDD might be significantly lower than the prescribed TDD. Otherwise, the initial rates could be too high and cause hypoglycemia. If there is suspicion that the patient might be frequently missing doses, use the weight-based method described below. Insulin-resistant patients, adolescent patients, and patients on low-carbohydrate diets may require higher basal amounts. Some clinicians use 40–60% of the TDD as basal insulin, and $0.5 \times TDD$ is widely used, though this has been recently refined to $0.47 \times TDD$ (Davidson 2008). Basal rates determined by continuous glucose monitoring have supported the lower rate of 40% (King 2010). Overreliance on basal insulin for glycemic control would be expected to lead to higher postprandial blood glucose levels and a greater tendency for hypoglycemia if meals are delayed. If the patient's recent glycemic control has been within desired target ranges, the TDD may need to be reduced 10–25% because most people require less insulin with pump therapy. If the TDD is not known, then a weight-based method (based on data with type 1 patients) should be used: $TDD = 0.24 \times$ body weight in pounds (Davidson 2008).

There are several methods for determining the starting basal rate. Unless you are certain of the exact hours the patient experiences either surges or decreases in blood glucose levels it is more straightforward to initiate pump therapy with one basal rate, and make changes as needed. Pump therapy initiation may reveal blood glucose elevations due to the dawn phenomenon. Pump therapy initiation may also reveal blood glucose reductions that differ in timing from what may have been assumed on MDI therapy. However, there are other factors that can contribute to high fasting blood glucose levels that might be misattributed to the dawn phenomenon. In overweight adults, or those with loud snoring, undiagnosed or untreated sleep apnea should certainly be considered (Pillai 2011; Harsch 2004). Though the association of sleep apnea and hyperglycemia is better established in type 2 diabetes, there is no reason to believe that blood glucose control in type 1 patients would not be adversely affected by untreated sleep apnea. Inconsistent a.m. hyperglycemia could also be due to dietary factors, such as high-fat meals, which can cause the blood glucose to increase in a delayed manner (Jones 2005). In that case, setting an increased early a.m. basal rate intended to correct the dawn phenomenon would be inappropriate.

## Method 1 (preferred by many clinicians)

1. Determine the patient's TDD by adding all doses of rapid- and intermediate- or long-acting insulin together.
2. Calculate 40% of the TDD and divide by 24. This calculation yields an hourly starting basal rate.
3. Reduce rate by 10% if the patient has blood glucose levels in range before starting on the pump.

*Example*

1. TDD: 34 units (5 units insulin glulisine before breakfast and before evening meal + 10 units a.m. NPH + 14 units bedtime (HS) NPH = 34 units total)
2. 34 units × 0.4 = 13.6 units ÷ 24 hour (h) = 0.56. The starting basal rate is 0.5 units/h (or 0.55 units/h if pump can be programmed in twentieth-unit increments) × 24 h.
3. If well controlled pre-pump, start at 0.4 or 0.45 units/h, which would be 10% lower than the calculated value.

## Method 2

1. Determine the patient's TDD by adding all doses of rapid- and intermediate- or long-acting insulin together.
2. Calculate 75–90% of the TDD. Use one-half of this amount and divide by 24. This calculation yields an hourly starting basal rate.

*Example 1*

1. TDD: 34 units (5 units insulin lispro before breakfast and before evening meal + 10 units a.m. NPH + 14 units HS NPH = 34 units total)
2. 34 units × 0.75 = 25.5 units ÷ 2 = 12.75 ÷ 24 h = 0.53. The starting basal rate is 0.5 units/h (or 0.55 units/h if pump can be programmed in twentieth-unit increments) × 24 h.

*Example 2*

1. TDD: 34 units (5 units insulin aspart before breakfast and before evening meal + 10 units a.m. NPH + 14 units hs NPH = 34 units total)

2. 34 units × 0.90 = 30.6 units ÷ 2 = 15.3 ÷ 24 h = 0.64. The starting basal rate is 0.6 units/h (or 0.65 units/h if pump can be programmed in twentieth-unit increments) × 24 h.

## Method 3

1. If using multiple doses of rapid-acting insulin with one dose of insulin glargine or insulin detemir, use the dose of insulin glargine or insulin detemir as the basal dose for the pump.
2. Divide the total dose of insulin glargine or insulin detemir by 24. This calculation yields an hourly starting basal rate.
3. If well-controlled pre-pump, reduce the calculated basal rate by 10–20%.

*Example*
1. Dose of insulin glargine = 20 units.
2. 20 units ÷ 24 h = 0.83. Starting basal rate is 0.8 or 0.85 units/h × 24 h.
3. If well-controlled pre-pump, reduce by 10–20%, so start at 0.7 units/h.

## Method 4

1. Use the weight-based method when accurate TDD data is not available, such as for a newly diagnosed patient, or a patient who misses a significant proportion of their doses: 0.24 × weight in pounds = TDD
2. TDD × 0.47 ÷ 24 hours = starting hourly basal rate.

*Example*
1. Type 1 diabetes patient, TDD not known, weight 145 lb.
2. 0.24 × 145 lb = 34.8; use as TDD
3. 34.8 × 0.47 = 16.4 units ÷ 24 hours = 0.68 units per hour; round to 0.6 or 0.65 or 0.675 units per hour.

Be conservative in implementing the starting rate if recent glucose records reveal frequent hypoglycemia. Initiate a rate slightly lower (by 0.1 or 0.05) than what was calculated. Increase the calculated rate slightly if recent blood glucose levels have been consistently elevated (>200 mg/dl). One leveling technique is to calculate starting basal rates using more than one method. Results are compared and averaged, or the lowest basal rate calculated is used.

# Calculating Insulin-to-Carbohydrate Ratios

A patient's insulin-to-carbohydrate ratio reflects his or her sensitivity to insulin. Generally, the more sensitive a person is to insulin, the higher the insulin-to-carbohydrate ratio. A patient in whom 1 unit of insulin covers 20 grams (g) carbohydrate is more insulin sensitive than a patient in whom 1 unit of insulin covers 12 g carbohydrate. Also, because some people are more or less insulin resistant at different times of day or have different levels of activity during the day, they may need to work with more than one ratio. The most common example is that patients may need more insulin to cover carbohydrate in the morning due to the dawn phenomenon.

Insulin-to-carbohydrate ratios are best determined by the RD/CDE during the carbohydrate counting teaching process or can be provided to the patient as a starting point by the prescribing physician or CDE. Pump manufacturers may also offer the services of a company-employed/per diem CDE to determine insulin-to-carbohydrate ratio and insulin correction/sensitivity factor calculations.

The ratios can be calculated with one of the methods described below. Use whichever method seems most appropriate based on the information you have available. It is a good idea to use one method to determine the insulin-to-carbohydrate ratio and another method to validate the ratio. These figures only represent a starting point and will likely need adjustment.

## Method 1: Food diary, insulin bolus dose, and SMBG information

This method is based on the amount of insulin currently used to cover consumed carbohydrate. Ask the patient to keep 3–7 days of records, including:

1. Fasting, preprandial, and 2-h PPG results
2. Preprandial insulin doses
3. Amount of carbohydrate consumed at meals and other times. It is helpful if the patient consumes the same amount of carbohydrate at each breakfast for the week, same amount of carbohydrate at each lunch for the week, etc., until the meal ratio is established.
4. Amount of all foods and beverages consumed, because fat, alcohol, and excessive protein (>4 oz/serving) may affect PPG levels

With these records, determine the amount of insulin the patient used to cover the carbohydrate consumed at each meal by dividing the total grams of carbohydrate by the number of units of insulin (Warshaw 2008).

*Example*

    Consumed 60 g carbohydrate

    Used 5 units rapid-acting insulin

    2-h PPG was within target range

    $60 \div 5 = 12$

    Insulin-to-carbohydrate ratio = 1:12

    1 unit of insulin covers 12 g carbohydrate

This method is most effective if SMBG records indicate that the patient is usually within his or her PPG targets. If blood glucose is generally not in control and carbohydrate intake is varied, this method will be less useful because frequent adjustments will be needed. This method may not practical for some patients, as the patient must be willing to keep detailed dietary intake and SMBG records. There are many smartphone applications (apps) that can be used to help a patient keep records of foods consumed, carbohydrate content, and doses taken.

## Method 2: The rule of 500 or 450 (Scherr 2009; Warshaw 2008)

This rule of thumb, widely used by clinicians to determine the insulin-to-carbohydrate ratio, is based on total (i.e., basal and bolus) daily insulin dose (TDD). The TDD is divided into 500 or 450 and the result is the amount of carbohydrate that 1 unit of rapid-acting insulin will cover, bringing blood glucose into the target range about 3–4 h after the meal. Many clinicians use the rule of 450 as a starting point for most patients (Scherr 2009).

*Example*

    TDD is 36 units

    Glucose levels are generally within or close to target range

    $450 \div 36 = 12.5$ (round up to 13)

    Insulin-to-carbohydrate ratio is 1:13

    1 unit of insulin covers 13 g carbohydrate

    OR

$500 \div 36 = 13.8$ (round up to 14)

Insulin-to-carbohydrate ratio is 1:14

1 unit of insulin covers 14 g carbohydrate

Data using continuous glucose monitoring suggests using a figure of 300 (King 2010), although this may be more aggressive than most clinicians use.

### Method 3: Using a formula based on body weight and TDD

Using this method, multiply the person's body weight (BW) in pounds by 2.8 and then divide the result by the TDD, giving the formula (BW) × 2.8 ÷ TDD = insulin-to-carbohydrate ratio. Of note, Davidson and associates found that the weight-based method was a significantly better predictor of the actual ICR in a group of well-controlled patients compared to using the Method 2 type of approach, so they do not recommend using the "450/500 rule" (Davidson 2008).

*Example*

TDD is 36 units

BW is 145 pounds

Glucose levels are generally within or close to target range

125 × 2.8 ÷ 36 = 11.3

Insulin-to-carbohydrate ratio is 1:12 (rounded up)

1 unit of insulin covers 12 g carbohydrate

### Method 4: Using the CF to calculate the ICR

Once a person's CF is calculated (see section below, Calculation of CF), multiplying the CF by 0.33 is another way to calculate an ICR (Warshaw 2008).

*Example 1*

CF is 60 mg/dl

60 × 0.33 = 19.8 (round to 20)

Insulin-to-carbohydrate ratio is 1:20

1 unit of insulin covers 20 g carbohydrate

*Example 2*

CF is 50 mg/dl

50 × 0.33 = 16.5 (round to 17)

Insulin-to-carbohydrate ratio is 1:17

1 unit of insulin covers 17 g carbohydrate

*Example 3*

CF is 45 mg/dl

$45 \times 0.33 = 14.8$ (round to 15)

Insulin-to-carbohydrate ratio is 1:15

1 unit of insulin covers 15 g carbohydrate

## Other Considerations

Deriving the ICR by the above methods is merely a starting point. Using differ-ent methods with the same parameters yields different results, so some clini-cians calculate the ICR using the average of two or three methods.

Some clinicians begin by assuming an ICR of 1:15 for most lean-to-average adults, 1:10 for insulin-resistant or overweight adults, and 1:20 or 1:25 for most children, who tend to be more insulin sensitive, but this method will likely underestimate the correct rate. If one is trying to minimize calcula-tions and wants to start with "ballpark" estimates, use the TDD (using the rule of 450) to more precisely estimate a reasonable starting point by know-ing that a patient with a TDD of 30 units will need an ICR of 1:15, one with a TDD of 45 units will need an ICR of 1:10, and a TDD of 60 units will need an ICR of 1:7.5.

Detailed records of SMBG results, carbohydrate intake, and insulin doses provide useful information to make ratio adjustments. Some patients may need different ratios for different times of the day, but this is best determined after the basal rates are correctly calculated and fine-tuned. And women may need differ-ent ratios at different phases of their menstrual cycle. Remind patients they will need to recalculate their ICR and use their new ratio if:

- Total daily dose of insulin changes by more than 10%
- Body weight changes by more than 3 to 5%
- There are lifestyle changes, such as a change in exercise, stress, or work hours
- There is significant illness or changes in medications known to affect blood glucose levels, particularly the use of oral glucocorticoids or a glucocorticoid injection into a joint
- They become pregnant, which necessitates an immediate evaluation and readjustment of insulin doses, monitoring schedule, diet, and follow-up requirements

# Calculating the Correction Factor (CF)

The insulin correction (or sensitivity) factor is the amount of blood glucose (in mg/dl) reduced by 1 unit of rapid-acting insulin over 3–4 h. The most widely used formula used to calculate the CF is 1700 divided by the TDD (Davidson 2008), although a recent CGM-based report suggested 1500 (King 2010). Whichever number is used will need to be adjusted for individual patients, and different CFs may be necessary for the same patient at different times of the day, something modern smart pumps allow. Consider that it may be safer to use a less aggressive setting at bedtime in order to reduce the risk of nocturnal hypoglycemia, which can result from an overcorrection of a bedtime high blood glucose reading.

The rules calculate the CF by dividing either 1700 or 1500 by the TDD.

*Example 1 (using 1700)*
   TDD is 34 units
   1700 ÷ 34 = 50
   CF is 50 mg/dl.
   One unit of rapid-acting insulin decreases blood glucose 50 mg/dl.

*Example 2 (using 1500)*
   TDD is 34 units
   1500 ÷ 34 = 44
   CF is 44 mg/dl.
   One unit of rapid-acting insulin decreases blood glucose 44 mg/dl

For patients with a history of hypoglycemia, or in patients for whom there is higher concern about the risk of hypoglycemia, increasing the calculated figure by 25–50% would be a more conservative way to start. The result could then be adjusted downward if needed. For example, if the calculated result is a CF of 50 mg/dl, start the patient with a CF of 75 mg/dl. As with all calculated insulin factors, these figures represent starting points and will need to be adjusted based on individual results.

# Calculating a Meal Bolus

After the insulin-to-carbohydrate ratio(s) and correction factor(s) have been established, meal and snack bolus doses can be calculated. You may want to provide written examples for the patient to review and, along with his or her

ICR(s) and CF(s), use these to practice. Most patients should be encouraged to use the smart pump features routinely, rather than calculate it themselves, but it is important that they understand how the pump calculates their dose so they know how much insulin to give if their pump breaks or malfunctions.

*Example*

    Glucose target is 110 mg/dl

    Insulin-to-carbohydrate ratio is 1:15

    CF is 50 mg/dl

    Pre lunch glucose is 187 mg/dl

| Item | Carbohydrate (g) |
|---|---|
| 1 turkey sandwich on rye bread | |
| (3 oz turkey = 0 g; 2 slices bread = 30 g) | 30 |
| 1 medium apple | 25 |
| 8 oz 1% milk | 12 |
| **Total** | **67** |

    Insulin needed to cover carbohydrate in the meal is 67 ÷ 15 = 4.46 units (round to 4.5)

    Insulin needed to return 187 mg/dl glucose to target is 187 − 110 = 77 mg/dl over target ÷ 50 = 1.54 units (round to 1.5)

    4.5 + 1.5 = 6.0 units for total premeal bolus

*Example*

    Glucose target is 100 mg/dl

    ICR is 1:18

    CF is 70 mg/dl

    Predinner glucose is 204 mg/dl

| Item | Carbohydrate (g) |
|---|---|
| 3 oz baked chicken | 0 |
| 1/2 cup mashed potatoes | 15 |
| 1 small dinner roll | 15 |
| 1 cup tossed salad | (5; do not need to count) |
| 1/2 cup broccoli | 5 |
| 2 Tbsp salad dressing | (<1; do not need to count) |
| 3/4 cup fresh pineapple chunks | 15 |
| **Total** | **50** |

Insulin needed to cover carbohydrate in meal is 50 ÷ 18 = 2.77 units (round to 2.8)

Insulin needed to return 204 mg/dl glucose to target is 204 − 100 = 104 mg/dl over target ÷ 70 = 1.48 units (round to 1.5)

2.8 + 1.5 = 4.3 units for total premeal bolus

# Identifying, Managing, and Preventing Hyperglycemia

Hyperglycemia, i.e., out-of-target values, can be troublesome, or severe enough to cause DKA. Discuss with the patient which hyperglycemic values necessitate an insulin adjustment and what situation constitutes a hyperglycemic crisis.

If the patient experiences hyperglycemia, the first step is to eliminate the possibility of any technical problems with the pump. Each insulin pump manufacturer provides basic guidelines for troubleshooting the technical aspects and functions of the pump that can lead to hyperglycemia, including, but not limited, to:

- loose Luer-lock connections
- air bubbles in the tubing
- cracked infusion set tubing
- dislodged or partially dislodged infusion set or pod
- selection of an ineffective infusion site, especially sites that have been used too frequently and may have developed scar tissue or lipohypertrophy
- site irritation or infection
- empty pump cartridge/reservoir
- expired or spoiled insulin
- incorrect bolus calculation
- missed bolus doses, which can be established by checking the pump memory in modern smart pumps
- incorrectly programmed basal rates
- leaving the pump in suspend mode for more than two hours

Note that infusion tubing is double-layered and has an inner core that carries the insulin. Even tying knots in the tubing will not impede the insulin flow. It must be emphasized that, unless there is a clear reason for the high blood glucose, such as a missed bolus or leaving the pump on "suspend" for several hours, **the infusion site or pod must be changed.** An infusion set can be partially dislodged and this may not be evident until after the cannula has been removed. This is less likely with an infusion set that allows visualization of the infusion site, but it can still occur. Trying to correct hyperglycemia with the insulin pump that resulted from a defective site will lead to worsening hyperglycemia and can result in ketoacidosis.

If the pump and infusion site are functioning properly, then the patient must correct the hyperglycemia with a dose of insulin. To calculate the amount of insulin needed to return blood glucose to within the desired target range, patients need to know three factors:

■ their target level
■ how much their glucose is above the target level
■ their correction factor (CF)

*Example*
> Target glucose level is 100 mg/dl
> Glucose is 264 mg/dl
> 264 mg/dl – 100 mg/dl = 164 mg/dl above target level
> CF is 55 mg/dl
> 164 mg/dl ÷ 55 mg/dl = 2.9 units
> The correction dose of insulin is 2.9 units using an insulin pump (3 units if using a syringe or insulin pen)

If a correction is needed just before a meal, teach the patient to add the amount of insulin calculated for the correction dose to the amount of insulin needed to cover the carbohydrate he or she is about to eat.

*Example*
> First, calculate the correction dose:
> Preprandial glucose level is 226 mg/dl
> Target glucose level is 100 mg/dl
> 226 mg/dl – 100 mg/dl = 126 mg/dl
> CF is 55 mg/dl
> 126 mg/dl ÷ 55 mg/dl = 2.3 units insulin to decrease the high preprandial glucose level

Next, calculate the dose needed to cover the meal:

    60 g carbohydrate are to be consumed

    Insulin-to-carbohydrate ratio is 1:15

    $60 \div 15 = 4$ units insulin to cover the carbohydrate

Then, add the two doses together:

    2.3 units + 4 units = 6.3 units insulin (insulin pump bolus) or round down to 6 units insulin if using syringe or pen

When using the CF for a manual calculation, it is important that the high blood glucose level being corrected to preprandial target range is actually the preprandial blood glucose and not a glucose measurement taken 1–2 h after the last meal. A blood glucose measurement 1–2 h after a meal reflects the action of the previous pre-meal dose of rapid-acting insulin, which is not yet complete. Smart insulin pumps can be enabled to use an "insulin on board" function to provide an estimate of how much insulin action is likely to occur from prior boluses, i.e., the "insulin on board." The pump takes into account this amount of insulin "on board" and subtracts it from the calculated/recommended correction bolus (see page 113). If the PPG result were to be used to calculate a correction dose using a preprandial target, the insulin bolus doses will overlap and lead to postprandial hypoglycemia, a process referred to as "stacking." If a pump patient is calculating his/her hyperglycemia dose manually (i.e., using a syringe or pen device instead of their pump), encourage the patient to make sure the dose they are calculating is based on the true preprandial blood glucose. For manual doses, provide instructions regarding specific insulin dose correction times. A reasonable recommendation for manual dosing would be to cut the calculated dose in half if the blood glucose was 2 hours postprandial to account for insulin action that is still on board.

Some clinicians prefer to have patients correct hyperglycemia using an algorithm, but this method tends to be less precise unless the patient is willing to calculate to fractions of units. Using an algorithm, the patient calculates a PPG correction dose beginning with the preprandial glucose/PPG target. For

"Duration of insulin action" OR "insulin on board" default pump settings are usually 3 or 4 hours.

example: bolus 1 unit of insulin for every 50 mg over 125 mg/dl at 3–4 h after eating. Patients may also find it easier to remember, "1 unit of insulin lowers my blood glucose ____ mg/dl" and to calculate an insulin dose using their individual CF.

Algorithm methods result in corrections that are not as precise as those calculated using a specific CF; they also require the patient to memorize their algorithm list or formula, or carry it with them at all times. This should be a backup to the pump. Pump therapy provides an opportunity to be more exact with insulin dosage, and patients should be encouraged to use the smart pump features if they are available. An advantage of using smart pump features is that it forces the patient to consider the two most important factors in determining a bolus amount: where the blood glucose is now, and what is going to be eaten. By doing so, it is less likely that the patient will be taking short cuts and bolusing fixed doses. Because a smart pump applies the different bolus factors in a consistent manner, it makes it easier to determine if the current settings are correct.

Another important issue in the management of hyperglycemia is the use of ketone test strips. Ask the patient to buy blood or urine ketone test strips, make sure the strips have not passed the expiration date, and know when and how to use them. Although ketone test strips are available over-the-counter, your patient may request or require a prescription for insurance reimbursement. Blood ketone strips require a meter.

Repeated episodes or a pattern of hyperglycemia require adjusting the basal rate(s), ICR, or CF. Looking for patterns, or pattern management, is an important tool to help sort out what setting needs to be adjusted. It is a good idea to reassess whether the patient is carbohydrate counting, and that they are doing it correctly. If the patient's carbohydrate counting is accurate, high blood glucose readings within 2 hours after a meal mean the bolus factors (ICR and CF) are likely at fault, and after 4 hours, the basal rate starts to be more important. However, if the bolus amounts are too low, such that the blood glucose is still too high after 3–4 hours, then the basal rate by itself will bring the glucose level back into the target range only slowly even if the rate is properly set. It should be noted that if a patient has daytime hyperglycemia and eats three meals a day that contain carbohydrate, most of the administered insulin during the day should be coming from the boluses, since the bolus amount should be 50–60% of the TDD, and it is usually mostly given over a period of 12–14 hours, versus the 20–25% of TDD that typically comes from the basal during the same time period. Therefore, it is crucial to set the bolus settings correctly in order to control daytime blood glucose levels. For more discussion of follow-up for pump patients, including performing basal rate checking and adjustment of the ICR(s) and CF(s), please refer to Chapter 6.

# Identifying, Managing, and Preventing Hypoglycemia

Hypoglycemia is the limiting factor in any intensive glucose management in both type 1 and insulin-requiring type 2 diabetes patients (Cryer 2002). Because blood glucose is kept much closer to target, whether by MDI or insulin pump therapy, there is less of a "glucose buffer" against hypoglycemia. Studies of insulin pumps versus MDI using older basal insulins in patients with type 1 diabetes showed much lower rates of hypoglycemia in patients using insulin pumps (Bode 1996; Boland 1999). There are few studies comparing MDI with basal insulin analogs to insulin pumps, and the rates of severe hypoglycemia were low in those studies in both groups, but in two studies there was better glucose control with less variability with insulin pumps (Doyle 2004, Hirsch 2005). Since studies of basal insulin analogs versus NPH have not shown a reduction in severe hypoglycemia rates, insulin pump therapy may still be considered the best therapeutic option to reduce the risk of hypoglycemia, especially severe hypoglycemia, in addition to reducing glucose variability and A1C and improving quality of life in patients with type 1 diabetes (Pickup 2008). In addition, patients who have serious problems with hypoglycemia on either MDI or pump therapy should be prescribed continuous glucose monitoring (Klonoff 2011).

Education in hypoglycemia management includes a review of basic guidelines, a glucagon prescription, and instructions on using glucagon for the patient's family members, friends, and/or significant other(s). This information should not be new to the patient or to the people around him or her. For mild to moderate hypoglycemia, teach and emphasize the Rule of 15:

■ Treat hypoglycemia with 15 g fast-acting carbohydrate
■ Check blood glucose after 15 minutes
■ Repeat the treatment as needed

Remind the patient that overtreatment of hypoglycemia may create a vicious cycle of low blood glucose followed by high blood glucose, which requires additional bolus doses, etc., with potential for subsequent weight gain. It is also important to emphasize that overtreatment of a low blood glucose reaction will generally not correct the hypoglycemia more quickly, it will just make the blood glucose go higher afterward. A general rule of thumb is that two or more unexplained instances of hypoglycemia in a week should prompt adjustments in basal rate(s), insulin-to-carbohydrate ratios, correction factor, or a combination of these parameters.

Hypoglycemia that occurs within 3 hours of a bolus is generally related to the bolus, whereas hypoglycemia that occurs more than 5 hours after the last bolus is likely a result of the basal rate being too high, but there are many other factors to consider. For example, exercise right after a bolus can cause hypoglycemia even if all the parameters are properly set, and can cause delayed hypoglycemia many hours later, even if the basal rate that is being used is correct for times when there was not exercise. Unusual increased activity, such as walking more than normal, or doing yard work over a prolonged period, could cause delayed hypoglycemia. High-fat food slows the absorption of carbohydrate, so the correct bolus amount may have been given, but the timing of the bolus needs to be changed to avoid postprandial hypoglycemia. In that case, a split bolus is needed, giving some insulin immediately and some as a delayed infusion, an approach that is easy with an insulin pump.

# Follow-Up Instructions

The patient should perform a glucose check and administer a bolus, if necessary, to correct hyperglycemia at the end of the pump start-up training. The prescribing physician and/or CDE should give the patient specific instructions for follow-up and management during the first few weeks after pump start-up (see Chapters 6 and 8). These include:

■ Perform SMBG initially a minimum of six times per day (3:00 a.m., fasting, before each meal, and bedtime) and record results. Additional postprandial checks at 2–3 h are also useful, and many patients actually add these glucose checks to their regimen. If, after a few days, a dawn phenomenon is detected and a compensatory basal rate adjustment is made and verified, the 3:00 a.m. check becomes unnecessary.

■ Record grams of carbohydrate consumed and specific food and beverage portions. This routine is especially helpful in identifying correct meal and snack bolus doses.

■ Avoid alcohol; high-fat foods, such as pizza, cakes, pies, some snack products, and some ethnic meals, including Italian, Mexican, and Chinese; and foods not usually consumed. Remind the patient to stick with a "basic" diet or "plain foods" and eliminate any food that could adversely cause erratic glucose levels. Reassure the patient that this is a temporary dietary adjustment during pump therapy initiation.

■ Avoid moderate to strenuous exercise for the first 2 weeks or until the basal rates, ICR, and CF are established.

■ Record all bolus doses using the ICR for meals and snacks and any CF bolus doses given for hyperglycemia, or use the smart pump feature if pump downloading is to be done. Some clinicians choose to delay use of the CF until the basal rates have been established because a correction bolus can lower blood glucose readings. If the correct basal rates have not been established, the clinician will not know if the basal insulin or the bolus dose is causing glucose fluctuations. Separate basal checks can also be done to determine the appropriateness of the basal rate(s), allowing use of the CF from the start. The CF dose should always be delivered if the patient is symptomatically hyperglycemic.

■ Record any unexpected or unusual events that could affect blood glucose levels, e.g., stress or illness, as well as the onset of menses.

■ Call in, fax, or e-mail the information to the clinician/CDE daily initially, then less frequently as allowed by the results. Downloading the pump to an internet-based smart pump data management system, if available, is also an option. Emphasize to the patient to enter all information in the smart pump using the appropriate features, if available. Provide the patient with specific names, numbers, and times to reach the clinician/CDE. Call the clinician/CDE for assistance with glycemic control or illness.

Call the pump manufacturer support service with any questions or problems related to the technical functions of the pump if they cannot be answered by the clinician/CDE.

A patient may require a follow-up visit within 1 week to review and to observe an infusion set or pod site change and pump syringe/cartridge removal and new fill. Some clinicians/CDEs do this "as needed," whereas others schedule an automatic 1-week or "next site change" brief appointment. Family support is critical in the first few weeks after pump start-up, and including the new pump patient's family members and/or significant others in a meeting to review lifestyle issues during this time may be helpful.

The patient should schedule a return visit to the clinician 4–6 weeks after the pump start-up for a review of SMBG and insulin doses and inspection of infusion sites. Many patients feel empowered after initiating pump therapy and will delay or reschedule appointments with their physician and/or CDEs, saying, "I'm doing great on the pump. I don't need to see my doctor or educator right now." Although self-management at the highest levels of diabetes care is the goal, emphasize to the patient the importance of clinical monitoring of A1C quarterly (patients with type 1 diabetes) or at least biannually (patients with type 2 diabetes) and good communication with the healthcare team. Ask the pump patient to maintain a regular visit/appointment schedule with healtcare professionals to evaluate his or her level of control, glucose patterns, insulin doses, and the pump's features and options. An insulin pump is a wonderful diabetes management tool, but it is not a license for the patient to practice medicine, and even well-controlled patients often benefit from some fine-tuning. Once the patient becomes comfortable with the basics of the pump, encourage him/her to try to use some of the more advanced features, like extended/square wave and combination/dual wave bolus features for high-fat foods, temporary basal rates to prevent exercise induced hypoglycemia, etc. See Chapter 7, Other Considerations in Pump Therapy Management.

# Additional Considerations

## Diabetic Gastroparesis

Diabetic gastroparesis refers to chronic delayed gastric emptying, which increases in incidence with the duration of diabetes, is more common in type 1 diabetes, and is associated with poor glucose control and the presence of other diabetic complications. It is thought to be on the basis of impaired neural control of gastric function, which may be a manifestation of autonomic neuropathy. Variable blood glucose control complicates the assessment of gastroparesis because acute hyperglycemia causes delayed gastric emptying even in non-diabetic subjects. Suggestive symptoms include nausea, vomiting, early satiety, and post-meal bloating, but there is significant overlap with other causes of gastrointestinal symptoms, so confirmatory testing with emptying studies and endoscopy is necessary to make the diagnosis (Parkman 2004).

Gastroparesis complicates blood glucose management because it can be associated with a delayed nutrient absorption (Ishii 2004), which can lead to hypoglycemia within several hours of a rapid insulin analog meal dose, followed by hyperglycemia after 3–4 hours. Often patients will be afraid to take insulin for a meal due to fears of hypoglycemia, which causes them to run very high blood glucose levels. The use of an insulin pump in type 1 diabetes patients with severe gastroparesis has been shown to dramatically reduce the number of hospital days, reduce glycemic variability, and improve glycemic control (Sharma 2011).

Insulin pump therapy allows using a split meal bolus, which would be expected to lead to a better match between insulin pharmacokinetics and nutrient absorption. For example, splitting a bolus dose with 50% given immediately and 50% spread over the next 4–6 hours is one approach (See Chapter 7, Other Considerations in Pump Therapy Management). Continuous glucose monitoring is very useful in monitoring patients with gastroparesis and can help assure that the recommended timing of meal doses has the desired effect.

## Pramlintide

Healthy (i.e., non-diabetes) patients will rarely have a postprandial blood glucose level above 140 mg/dl (American Diabetes Association 2001), but patients with diabetes rarely achieve this degree of postprandial blood glucose control, even those who have an A1C below 7% (Schrot 2004). Use of CGM demonstrates that most insulin-requiring patients, even those with an A1C at or below goal, need significant alterations in therapy to achieve postprandial blood glucose control. Increasing the ICRs, increasing the time interval between delivering the bolus and eating to 15–20 minutes (Coory 2010), reducing carbohydrate intake, avoiding high-glycemic foods, and exercising after meals can all help lower postprandial blood glucose excursions. The use of pramlintide, a synthetic amylin analog, is another available option to reduce postprandial hyperglycemia and improve glycemic control.

Amylin is a naturally occurring glucoregulatory hormone that is co-secreted along with insulin from the pancreatic beta cells. To the extent that insulin secretion is deficient, amylin secretion is likewise deficient, since both insulin and amylin are released from the same beta-cell granules. Amylin affects the appearance of meal-derived glucose. In a glucose-dependent manner, amylin modulates appetite and food intake (delays gastric emptying) and reduces glucagon levels. Amylin itself is not a viable pharmacologic agent. Pramlintide is a synthetic amylin analog that reproduces all the physiologic effects of native amylin, leading to less postprandial hyperglycemia, but it has a pharmacology that allows therapeutic use by the administration of subcutaneous preprandial injections (Edelman 2002). Clinical studies with pramlintide have demonstrated that both type 1 (Ratner 2004; Levetan 2003) and type 2 (Hollander 2003) diabetes patients can achieve better blood glucose control with a lower A1C level without an increase in hypoglycemia and with modest weight loss.

Use of pramlintide administered as a preprandial injection in patients using an insulin pump should be considered when a patient has suboptimal blood glucose control, is having problems with weight gain, or both. Pramlintide must be administered by subcutaneous injection with a prefilled pen before each meal. *It should never be mixed with insulin in an insulin pump or insulin syringe.* Pramlintide is not approved for use in pregnant women, and is contraindicated in patients with gastroparesis (Amylin Pharmaceuticals 2008). While not contraindicated, it may not be well tolerated in patients with significant gastroesophageal reflux.

The risk of postprandial hypoglycemia, which would occur within 3 hours of injection, is potentially increased when using pramlintide, especially in patients with type 1 diabetes. Therefore, it is recommended that the bolus dose of insulin be reduced by 50% on initiation of pramlintide. However, a clinical study in type 1 patients showed the need for only a small reduction in insulin (3–6%) by the end of a 1-year trial (Ratner 2004), so it is very likely that a 50% bolus reduction may be too great. The insulin bolus dose could be initially reduced by 30–50% but rapidly titrated upward to achieve postprandial blood glucose control. Using this technique, the risk of postprandial hypoglycemia is low (Amylin Pharmaceuticals 2008). It is also clear that the blood glucose often starts to rise again after 3 hours from the delayed absorption of ingested nutrients, so the use of a split bolus or extended bolus may be beneficial to prevent hyperglycemia prior to the next meal. Use of a 50–70% bolus delivered immediately with 30–50% extended over 3 to 4 hours is a reasonable starting point.

The most common side effect of pramlintide is nausea, which is more of a problem in type 1 patients than in type 2 patients, probably because type 1 patients have a complete amylin deficiency, while a patient with type 2 diabetes who has any endogenous insulin secretion would still have some endogenous amylin. Nausea is usually mild to moderate and transient, and fades within the first month of therapy (Ratner 2004; Hollander 2003) and can be minimized by titrating the dose in a step wise fashion:

- Type 1 diabetes: Start at 15 mcg before meals containing at least 250 kcal or 30 g of carbohydrate, increase by 15 mcg increments as allowed by the resolution of nausea, up to 60 mcg. Some patients do not need to go up to the full 60 mcg dose.
- Type 2 diabetes: Start at 60 mcg before meals, increase to 120 mcg as allowed by the resolution of nausea.

In summary, pramlintide can help improve glycemic control in both type 1 and type 2 diabetes patients, principally by improving postprandial blood glucose levels, and potentially reducing appetite with an additional advantage of modest weight loss, but requires some trial and error as one adjusts the dose of insulin. For best control, pump patients should be encouraged to take advantage of the split bolus option offered by smart insulin pumps. Despite the package insert warning on hypoglycemia, the incidence of hypoglycemia in clinical trials is low.

## Use of U-500 Human Regular Insulin in an Insulin Pump

The obesity epidemic has led to a growing number of type 2 diabetic patients, and also higher insulin requirements in some of those patients. There are now more patients requiring very high doses of insulin (above 200 units a day), many of whom remain in suboptimal control. The growing number of type 2 diabetes patients requiring very high doses of insulin has spurred interest in the **off-label** (i.e., not approved by the U.S. Food and Drug Administration [FDA]) use of U-500 human regular insulin (U-500) in insulin pumps (Lane 2009; Reutrakul 2012).

As of this writing, all insulin except U-500 is only available in a concentration of 100 units per ml, or U-100. Use of high doses of U-100 insulin is problematic for several reasons. If administered by syringe, the need for more than 100 units at a time requires a second injection, and more than 60 to 80 units at a time requires a second injection if dosed via currently available insulin pens. The injection of the high volumes needed to give large doses as U-100 insulin can be more painful, which might decrease compliance, and there is also concern that the efficiency of absorption may be worsened with high-volume injections, which would worsen glucose control (Lane 2009). If very high doses of insulin are administered with a pump, the cost of supplies goes up markedly and practicality decreases, due to the need for more frequent site changes, which could reduce compliance. There may be a greater likelihood of site irritation and poor site absorption with very high doses (personal observation, Nicholas B. Argento, MD) as well, which would worsen glucose control.

Use of U-500 has been reported to significantly improve blood glucose control in type 2 diabetes patients requiring very high doses of insulin, whether administered via injection (Neal 2005) or via pump (Lane 2006; Lane 2010). One review reported an average A1C reduction of 1.4%, and little to no increase in hypoglycemia, though weight gain was reported. It was noted that there would be substantial cost savings versus high-dose injected insulin analog therapy, even taking into account the cost of pump therapy. There was not a consistent change in total insulin dose in the studies that have been published, most of which are small and many of which are observational (Lane 2009).

The pharmacology of U-500 at a low dose is closer to that of NPH insulin, with a reported onset of action of 45 minutes, a peak action at 7 to 8.5 hours, and duration of action of 11.5 hours (Khan 2009). At high dose in type 2 diabetes patients, the onset is within 1/2 hour, but with delayed peak activity (5 hours) and prolonged duration (Davidson 2010). When compared directly to high-dose U-100 human regular insulin in healthy obese subjects, U-500 had a similar onset by 30 minutes, but a delay to peak activity and prolonged duration of action, with activity lasting as long as 21.5 hours (de la Peña 2011). The slower onset of action compared to insulin analogs and long duration of action requires altering the usual dose recommendations for an insulin pump, as detailed below. U-500 should be given a half hour before eating when used as a bolus insulin.

Use of U-500, including in a pump, should be considered in the following types of patients (modified from Lane 2009):

■ Type 2 diabetes with severe insulin resistance
■ Insulin-requiring diabetes with a need for insulin above 200 units a day
■ High-dose glucocorticoid therapy

- Post-transplant associated severe insulin resistance
- Gestational or pregestational diabetes with severe insulin resistance
- Defects of insulin action
- Lipodystrophic diabetes, congenital or acquired
- Type A insulin resistance syndromes (leprechaunism and Rabson-Mendenhall syndrome)
- Rare forms of immune-mediated diabetes such as anti-insulin receptor antibodies (Type B insulin resistance syndrome)

Prescribing U-500 is more complex because there are no U-500 syringes and the current available insulin pumps assume the insulin used in the pump is in a concentration of U-100. When writing a prescription for U-500, the actual number of units must appear on the prescription. A prudent way to write a prescription for a syringe would be to specify the actual units, followed by what the number of units in a U-100 syringe will be and the volume. For example, to prescribe 50 units before each meal, write "50 units (10 units in a U-100 syringe, 0.1 cc/mL) before each meal" (Lane 2009). For a patient using an insulin pump who needs 350 units a day, write "350 units (0.35 mL) a day in insulin pump." Use of a U-500 instruction sheet with a dose conversion is very helpful. An example is in Chapter 8, Forms and Resources.

Determining starting rates with U-500 insulin in a pump depends on the total dose range and the patient's starting level of blood glucose control. Use of a pump for U-500 insulin is reasonable for patients who require between 150–600 units a day, though U-500 insulin is not FDA-approved for this use. For patients much above 600 units a day, a pump may be impractical. When calculating a patient's total daily dose, it is **vital to verify that the patient is actually taking the prescribed doses**, since patients do not always adhere fully to insulin recommendations. Reviewing the patient's injection technique and examining the patient's injection sites would also be important to verify that they are injecting properly.

Recommendations from Lane and associates on initial dosing are as follows: In general, a lower percentage of the daily insulin, 20–50%, should be given as the basal rate, since bolus doses of U-500 have a prolonged duration that in effect contribute to the basal rate. For patients who have an A1C below 8%, cutting the total daily dose by 10–20% is reasonable; for those with an A1C between 8–10%, no change in the initial total dose is recommended; for patients with an A1C above 10%, an increase of 10–20% is reasonable. A greater percentage of the bolus should be given at breakfast to reduce the risk of nocturnal hypoglycemia, with a proposed starting dose breakdown of 20–30% at breakfast and 15–25% at lunch and supper/evening meal (Lane 2009). Particular attention needs to be paid to the risk of nocturnal hypoglycemia in patients who carbohydrate count rather than giving fixed meal doses, because the prolonged duration of an often large dinner bolus can lead to high insulin levels at 2–3 a.m. Monitoring 2–3 a.m. blood glucose levels is a prudent measure when first starting a patient on U-500 insulin. It may be safer to give more of the basal rate during the waking hours initially in order to further minimize the risk of nocturnal hypoglycemia. For the same reason, it is best to not have patients on U-500 administer correction insulin before bed, at least initially.

Use of U-500 in an insulin pump versus the use of injections in a highly insulin-resistant patient with diabetes has many of the same advantages that a pump has in other patients, including improved ease of premeal doses, and thus possibly improved compliance, improved flexibility in adjusting basal doses, and the possibility of taking advantage of smart pump features to better guide dosing.

**It is very helpful to always talk about "pump units" to a patient on U-500 in a pump, after explaining that each "pump unit" will equal 5 units of insulin.** Anecdotal experience demonstrates that pump patients grasp this concept easily. However, it may be best for the HCP/prescriber her/himself to set the patient's smart pump settings because the effect of using U-500 on these settings can be confusing. It is important to keep straight how the different pump settings are affected by the use of U-500:

- **Basal rate: divide the desired actual rate by 5 to get the "pump unit" rate.** For example, if the desired actual basal rate is 5.5 units an hour, then divide 5.5 units an hour by 5 to set the "pump unit" rate as 1.1 units an hour.
- **Boluses: divide the desired actual number of units by 5 to get the "pump unit" dose.** For example, in a patient who was using a fixed premeal dose of 50 units, to give 50 units, the patient would enter 50 ÷ 5 = 10 "pump units" as a bolus.
- **Insulin correction/sensitivity factor (CF/ISF):** This number is entered into smart pumps, in most cases, as the amount of blood glucose lowered from 1 unit of insulin. For example if 1 unit lowers the blood glucose by 10

mg/dl, then the setting is 10. For a patient on U-500 insulin, that number would be the amount one would expect the blood glucose to fall with 5 units of insulin, since 1 pump unit (of U-500 insulin) = 5 units, so **multiply the factor by 5.** For example, if the patient has a correction/sensitivity factor of 10: correction/sensitivity setting of 10 × 5 (to correct for the number of units in 1 pump unit) = 50 as the correct CF/ISF setting—that is, 5 units = 1 pump unit that would be expected to lower the blood glucose by 50 mg/dl. (The patient should be cautioned to only cover premeal blood glucose levels and only if they had not bolused within 4 hours to avoid stacking correction doses, and not to cover bedtime readings, at least initially, to avoid causing nocturnal hypoglycemia.)

- **Insulin-to-carbohydrate ratio (ICR):** This is entered into most smart pumps as the number of grams of carbohydrate that will be covered by 1 unit of insulin. Since a pump unit (of U-500 insulin) is 5 units, multiply the ICR number × 5, since it would be the grams of carbohydrate covered by 5 units of insulin. For example, if 1 unit covers 2 grams of carbohydrate, then to convert to pump units, multiply 2 grams × 5 = 10 grams, which would mean 1 pump unit = 5 units would cover 10 grams of carbohydrate. The ICR would be set at 10. **Consider using fixed meal doses rather than carbohydrate counting in highly insulin-resistant individuals** (Lane 2009) in order to keep dosing simpler.
- **Duration:** best to set at 6 hours since the duration of action is so long.

*Examples*
1. Patient with an A1C of 9.2% on a TDD of 240 units of insulin daily to start on U-500 in an insulin pump with fixed doses at mealtimes.
   - Since the A1C is between 8 and 10%, no change in the initial TDD is recommended.
   - Basal rate: 240 units TDD: give 30% as basal: 0.30 × 240 units = 72 units as basal.
   - Divide 72 units by 24 hours = 3.0 units an hour × 24 hours; alternatively, adjust for a lower starting night basal by recommending that the basal be 2.5 units an hour from 9 PM to 5 a.m., and 3.2 units from 5 a.m. to 9 p.m. (preferred to reduce the risk of nocturnal hypoglycemia).
   - Set pump basal rates: Basal 9 p.m. to 5 a.m. is 2.5 units ÷ 5 = 0.5 pump units per hour; basal 5 AM to 9 PM is 3.2 units ÷ 5 = 0.64 pump units per hour, round to 0.65 pump units per hour.

- Bolus doses: 240 units TDD, give 70% as premeal boluses: 0.70 × 240 units = 168 units.
- Bolus dose 168 units: give 30% breakfast, 20% lunch, 20% supper: 0.30 × 168 units = 72 units before breakfast, 0.20 × 168 units = 48 units before lunch and supper, round off to 70 units and 50 units, respectively.
- Set pump bolus doses: Recommended meal boluses: 70 units before breakfast ÷ 5 = 14 pump units entered in as bolus; 50 units before lunch and supper ÷ 5 = 10 pump units entered as meal bolus before lunch and supper, plus CF(ISF) if needed.
- Target blood glucose: 120 mg/dl; duration of insulin: 6 hours
- Insulin correction/sensitivity factor: 1500 or 1700 ÷ TDD; will use 1700. 1700 ÷ 240 units = 7.1, but would round up to 8 as insulin CF/ISF.
- Set pump CF(ISF): 8 (calculated value) × 5 (to adjust for each pump unit being 5 units of insulin) = 40.

1. Patient with an A1C of 7.8%, on a TDD of 240 units daily, to start on U-500 in an insulin pump with carbohydrate counting.
   - Since the A1C is below 8%, will reduce the TDD by 15% TDD: 240 units × 0.85 = 204 units.
   - 204 units TDD, give 30% as basal: 0.30 × 204 units TDD = 61.2, round to 61 units over 24 hours.
   - Basal rate: Divide 61 units by 24 hours = 2.54 units, round to 2.5 units per hour × 24 hours; adjust for a lower starting night basal by recommending that the basal be 2.0 units an hour from 9 PM to 5 AM, and 2.75 units from 5 AM to 9 PM to reduce the risk of nocturnal hypoglycemia.
   - Set pump basal: basal 9 PM to 5 AM is 2.0 units ÷ 5 = 0.4 pump units per hour; basal 5 AM to 9 PM is 2.75 units ÷ 5 = 0.55 pump units per hour.
   - Insulin-to-carbohydrate ratio: 450 ÷ TDD = 450 ÷ 204 = 2.04, round to an ICR of 2.
   - Set pump ICR: ICR = 2 × 5 (to adjust for each pump unit containing 5 units of insulin) = 10 grams at breakfast and lunch. It would be prudent to use less insulin for carbohydrate consumed at supper/evening meal, at least initially, since the long duration of U-500 can lead to high insulin levels in the middle of the night, when the need for insulin tends to be lower. For supper, start at 3 grams actual = 15 grams as the ICR setting.
   - Target: 120 mg/dl; duration of insulin: 6 hours.

- Insulin correction/sensitivity factor: 1500 or 1700 ÷ TDD; will use 1700. 1700 ÷ 204 units = 8.3, but would round to 9 as CF/ISF.
- Set pump CF (ISF): 9 (calculated value) × 5 (to adjust for each pump unit being 5 units of insulin) = 45.

## Follow-up for U-500 pump patients

It is advisable to have the patient report their blood glucose results to the HCP within 24–48 hours of starting U-500 insulin, and to check blood glucose levels at 2–3 AM for at least the first week. Although on average, total insulin doses do not decrease in patients started on U-500 insulin (Lane 2009), there are certainly individual patients who will see a large drop in their blood glucose values almost immediately, perhaps because of improved efficiency of insulin absorption, or perhaps better adherence to prescribed dosing and closer attention to diet. Frequent SMBG or, better yet, ongoing CGM use is essential to detect patients who need a reduction in insulin doses.

Some of the highly insulin-resistant patients have been in poor glucose control for years and are quite discouraged before they start U-500. The successful use of U-500 insulin in a pump in such a patient is highly gratifying for both the HCP and the patient.

## REFERENCES

American Diabetes Association: Clinical practice recommendations. *Diabetes Care* 36:S11–S66, 2013

American Diabetes Association: Postprandial blood glucose. *Diabetes Care* 24:775–778, 2001

Amylin Pharmaceuticals, Inc.: SYMLIN (pramlintide acetate) injection [Prescribing Information]. San Diego, CA: Amylin Pharmaceuticals, Inc., 2005–2008

Bode BW, Steed RD, Davidson PC: Reduction in severe hypoglycemia with long-term continuous subcutaneous insulin infusion in type 1 diabetes. *Diabetes Care* 19:324–327, 1996

Boland EA, Grey M, Oesterle A, Fredrickson L, Tamborlane WV: Continuous subcutaneous insulin infusion: a new way to lower risk of severe hypoglycemia, improve metabolic control, and enhance coping in adolescents with type 1 diabetes. *Diabetes Care* 22:1779–1784, 1999

Cryer PE: Hypoglycaemia: the limiting factor in the glycaemic management of type I and type II diabetes. *Diabetologia* 45:937–948, 2002

Davidson MB, Navar MD, Echeverry D, Duran P: U-500 Regular Insulin. Clinical experience and pharmockinetics in obese, severely insulin-resistant type 2 diabetic patients. *Diabetes Care* 33:281–283, 2010

Davidson PC, Hebblewhite HR, Steed RD, Bode BW: Analysis of guidelines for basal-bolus insulin dosing: basal insulin, correction factor, and carbohydrate-to-insulin ratio. *Endocrine Practice* 14:1095–1101, 2008 de la Peña A, Riddle M, Morrow LA, Jiang HH, Linnebjerg H, Scott A, Win KM, Hompesch M, Mace KF, Jacobson JG, Jackson JA: Pharmacokinetics and pharmacodynamics of high-dose human regular U-500 insulin versus human regular U-100 insulin in healthy obese subjects. *Diabetes Care* 34:2496–2501, 2011

Doyle EA, Weinzimer SA, Steffen AT, Ahern JA, Vincent M, Tamborlane WV: A randomized, prospective trial comparing the efficacy of continuous subcutaneous insulin infusion with multiple daily injections using insulin glargine. *Diabetes Care* 27:1554–1558, 2004

Edelman SV, Weyer C: Unresolved challenges with insulin therapy in type 1 and type 2 diabetes: potential benefit of replacing amylin, a second *b*-cell hormone. *Diabetes Technol Ther* 4:175–189, 2002

Handelsman Y, Mechanick JI, Blonde L, Grunberger G, Bloomgarden ZT, Bray GA, Dagogo-Jack S, Davidson JA, Einhorn D, Ganda O, Garber AJ, Hirsch IB, Horton ES, Ismail-Beigi F, Jellinger PS, Jones KL, Jovanovic L, Lebovitz H, Levy P, Moghissi ES, Orzeck EA, Vinik AI, Wyne KL; AACE Task Force for Developing Diabetes Comprehensive Care Plan: American Association of Clinical Endocrinologists medical guidelines for developing a diabetes mellitus comprehensive care plan. *Endocrine Pract* 17:S1–S53, 2011

Harsch IA, Schahin SP, Radespiel-Tröger M, Weintz O, Jahreiss H, Fuchs FS, Wiest GH, Hahn EG, Lohmann T, Konturek PC, Ficker JH: Continuous positive airway pressure treatment rapidly improves insulin sensitivity in patients with obstructive sleep apnea syndrome. *Am J Respir Crit Care Med* 169:156–162, 2004

Hirsch IB, Bode BW, Garg S, Lane WS, Sussman A, Hu P, Santiago OM, Kolaczynski JW: Continuous subcutaneous insulin infusion (CSII) of insulin aspart versus multiple daily injections of insulin aspart/insulin glargine in type 1 diabetic patients previously untreated with CSII. *Diabetes Care* 28:533–538, 2005

Hollander PA, Levy P, Fineman MS, Maggs DG, Shen LZ, Strobel SA, Weyer C, Kolterman OG: Pramlintide as an adjunct to insulin therapy improves long-term glycemic and weight control in patients with type 2 diabetes: a 1 year randomized controlled trial. *Diabetes Care* 26:784–790, 2003

Ishii M, Nakamura T, Kasai F, Onuma T, Baba T, Takebe K: Altered postprandial insulin requirement in IDDM patients with gastroparesis. *Diabetes Care* 17:901–903, 1994

Jones SM, Quarry JL, Caldwell-McMillan M, Mauger DT, Gabbay RA: Optimal insulin pump dosing and postprandial glycemia following a pizza meal using the continuous glucose monitoring system. *Diab Technol Therap* 7:233–240, 2005

Khan M, Sarabu B: The pharmacokinetic and pharmacodynamic properties of regular U-500 insulin in healthy obese subjects. *Diabetes* 58:2333P, 2009

King AB: How much do I give? Reevaluation of insulin dosing estimation formulas using continuous glucose monitoring. *Endoc Pract* 16:428–432, 2010

Kitzmiller JL, Block JM, Brown FM, Catalano PM, Conway Dl, Coustan DR, Gunderson EP, Herman WH, Hoffman LD, Inturrisi M, Jovanovic LB, Kjos SI, Knopp RH, Montoro MN, Ogata ES, Paramsothy P, Reader DM, Rosenn BM, Thomas AM, Kirkman MS: Managing preexisting diabetes for pregnancy: summary of evidence and consensus recommendations for care. *Diabetes Care.* 31:1060–1079, 2008

Klonoff DC, Buckingham B, Christiansen JS, Montori VM, Tamborlane WV, Vigersky RA, Wolpert H: Continuous glucose monitoring: an Endocrine Society clinical practice guideline. *J Clinical Endocr Metabol* 96:2968–2979, 2011

Lane WS: Use of U-500 regular insulin by continuous subcutaneous insulin infusion in patients with type 2 diabetes and severe insulin resistance. *Endocr Pract* 12:251–256, 2006

Lane WS, Cochran EK, Jackson JA, Scism-Bacon JL, Corey IB, Hirsch IB, Skyler JS: High dose insulin therapy: is it time for U-500? *Endocr Pract* 15:71–79, 2009

Lane WS, Weinrib SL, Rappaport JM, Przestrzelski T: A prospective trial of U500 insulin delivered by Omnipod in patients with type 2 diabetes mellitus and severe insulin resistance. *Endocr Pract* 16:778–784, 2010

Levetan C, Want LL, Weyer C, Strobel SA, Crean J, Wang Y, Maggs DG, Kolterman OG, Chandran M, Mudaliar SR, Henry RR: Impact of pramlintide on glucose fluctuations and postprandial glucose, glucagon, and triglyceride excursions among patients with type 1 diabetes intensively treated with insulin pumps. *Diabetes Care* 26:1–8, 2003

Neal JM: Analysis of effectiveness of human U-500 insulin in patients unresponsive to conventional insulin therapy. *Endocr Pract* 11:305–307, 2005

Parkman HP, Hasler WL, Fisher RS: American Gastroenterological Association technical review on the diagnosis and treatment of gastroparesis. *Gastroenterology* 127:1592–1622, 2004

Pickup JC, Renard E: Long-acting insulin analogs versus insulin pump therapy for the treatment of type 1 and type 2 diabetes. *Diabetes Care* 31 (Suppl. 2):S140–S145, 2008

Pillai A, Warren G, Gunathilake W, Idris I: Effects of sleep apnea severity on glycemic control in patients with type 2 diabetes prior to continuous positive airway pressure treatment. *Diab Technol and Therap.* 13:945–949, 2011

Ratner RE, Dickey R, Fineman M, Maggs DG, Shen L, Strobel SA, Weyer C, Kolterman OG: Amylin replacement with pramlintide as an adjunct to insulin therapy improves long-term glycaemic and weight control in type 1 diabetes mellitus: a 1 year, ramdomized controlled trial. *Diabet Med* 21:1204–1212, 2004

Reutrakul S, Wroblewski K, Brown RL: Clinical use of U-500 regular insulin: review and meta-analysis. *J Diabetes Sci Technol* 6:412–20, 2012.

Sherr J, Tamborlane W, Bode B. Insulin pump therapy. In *Therapy for Diabetes Mellitus and Related Disorders, 5th ed.,* Lebowitz HE, ed. Alexandria, VA: American Diabetes Association. 2009.

Schrot RJ: Targeting plasma glucose: preprandial versus postprandial. *Clinical Diabetes* 22:169–172, 2004

Sharma D, Morrison G, Joseph F, Purewal TS, Weston PJ: The role of continuous subcutaneous insulin infusion therapy in patients with diabetic gastroparesis. *Diabetologia* 54:2768–2770, 2011

Warshaw HS, Bolderman KM: *Practical Carbohydrate Counting: A How-to-Teach Guide for Health Professionals, 2nd ed.* Alexandria, VA: American Diabetes Association, 2008

## CHAPTER 6

# Pump Therapy Management (Keeping Patients on the Pump)

P atients are "fine-tuned" when the basal rate(s) and bolus doses, determined using the insulin-to-carbohydrate ratio (ICR) and correction factor (CF), yield results within the patient's target glycemic levels. This outcome may take several weeks or longer. The patient needs to collect information, e.g., SMBG records, carbohydrate intake, and bolus doses, to assist the clinician in evaluating his or her status. Careful monitoring and detailed record keeping in the early stages of pump therapy, although tedious, are necessary and beneficial.

The management of pump therapy requires assessing, evaluating, and modifying the basal rates, ICRs, and CF. When making changes with the patient, explain why and how adjustments are made. Your explanations will help increase the patient's understanding of the basics of pump therapy and build confidence in his or her ability to identify problems and practice appropriate self-management pump skills.

## Record Keeping

Explain to the new pump patient that a record ("log book") of SMBG results, carbohydrate intake, bolus doses (both meal and correction), and notes or comments about everyday events, such as exercise, illness, stress, alcohol intake, and onset of menses, is extremely helpful in determining changes that should be made. These changes include adjustments in the patient's basal rates or pump parameters, including ICRs and CFs.

There are several ways to obtain the patient's SMBG results ("log book"). A smart pump can store data entered by the patient, including SMBG values, food boluses, correction boluses, etc. You can direct the patient to return to your office several days after the pump start with their downloadable smart pump, downloadable glucose meter, or "paper" records in hand. Other options to retrieve a patient's data include a smart phone download, email, telephone call, or facsimile (fax).

# Using Pump Data

Pump software is available and provides information for the user, as well as the clinician, to review up to several months of data. But the data that is downloaded is only valuable if the pump user inputs as much information as possible, i.e. carb intake, blood glucose readings, basal rate changes, food/meal boluses, correction boluses, etc. Encourage the new pump patient to use the pump's features to capture as much data as possible. Not only will bolus doses be recorded, but the time of the doses will be visible and will aid in detecting glucose and intake patterns and trends. Additionally, other "patterns" can also be detected, such as behavior patterns, including when the patient changes basal rates, the infusion set, etc.

# Using Blood Glucose Meter Data

Many glucose meters store BG results and allow the user to retrieve the data in a number of ways, including scrolling through the results, value-by-value, or clicking on buttons to review an average of the values ranging from several days to several months. Some meters offer the ability to store insulin doses, exercise minutes, carbohydrate grams consumed, and other data pertinent to the BG result. Patterns of glucose control, e.g., low values at specific times of day, can also be identified using some BG meters.

Meters can be downloaded by patients at home or the HCP can download a patient's meter in the office, provided you have the meter-specific software and connection cable. There are also meters that can link to an insulin pump, thus eliminating the step to download the meter and compare the data to information stored in the pump.

Encourage your new pump patient to be diligent about performing SMBG often during pump therapy initiation. The more information you have regarding the patient's SMBG values, the better equipped you are to make adjustments to the patient's basal rates, ICRs, and CFs.

# Using Continuous Glucose Monitor Data

A continuous glucose monitor (CGM) system consists of a disposable transcutaneous glucose sensor connected to a transmitter that wirelessly sends glucose readings to a monitor/receiver. The sensor is inserted similarly to an insulin pump infusion set. The receiver can be a separate device or can actually be part of the pump, depending on the manufacturer. The screen on the receiver or pump displays the glucose level, along with graphic representations of the BG levels and arrows that indicate the direction and rate of change in the glucose concentration. A CGM sensor measures interstitial glucose every five minutes and then transmits the readings to the receiver or insulin pump. CGM sensors currently require a warm-up period and calibration with the patient's BG meter at least twice/day. There are several brands, including 3-day and 7-day sensors. A CGM sensor does not eliminate the need for SMBG conducted with a BG meter. Due to the lag time of up to 20 minutes between the BG and interstitial glucose level, a sensor reading taken alone is not accurate enough to make a decision about a bolus insulin dose. The U.S. Food and Drug Administration has recommended that patients continue to use their blood glucose meters to confirm sensor readings and before making a decision about dosing insulin (U.S. FDA 2013).

Depending on the manufacturer, integrated insulin pump data and sensor data can be downloaded to a secure website that is accessible by the HCP. This feature may be useful in reviewing a patient's data before or between the patient's appointments.

A CGM system provides pump users with continuous BG data, including readings and trends, as well as alerts and alarms. But patients may become overwhelmed with the amount of data generated by a glucose sensor, especially during pump therapy initiation. If the patient has used a CGM system prior to pump initiation and is comfortable with the interpretation of readings and trends, a CGM system is a useful tool, along with the patient's SMBG values, to identify patterns and make decisions about meal and correction boluses and/or adjusting basal rates. For example, when determining or changing a basal rate and the patient's SMBG values are within target, but the CGM data indicates a rising trend, consider an increase in the basal rate. If the patient is about to eat, and the SMBG value is within target but the CGM data reveals a decreasing trend, the patient may consider a reduction in the ICR (resulting in a lower meal bolus [King 2012]).

Using a CGM system can be useful during pump therapy, but patient education is key in achieving success. Learn the patient's schedule to decide the most appropriate times to insert and calibrate a sensor. The patient's target BG levels should be set so that alarms do not occur frequently (e.g., slightly above desired targets). Alarms for projected glucose and threshold glucose levels are best set in stages so that the patient does not experience frustration with repeated alarms throughout the day. Review the pharmacologic action of insulin and remind the patient not to perform frequent correction boluses. Studies have demonstrated that the use of sensor-augmented pump therapy can result in an increase in the number of boluses (Racah 2009; Rigla 2008). The pump's "insulin-on-board" feature will assist in making decisions about a correction bolus and prevent "stacking" of insulin.

Hypoglycemia and hyperglycemia events can be better anticipated and managed with the use of a glucose sensor; thus sensor-augmented insulin pump therapy can help improve glycemic control (Buse 2012, Bergenstal 2010). An insulin pump that is paired with a CGM can actually suspend insulin delivery after a preset glycemic threshold has been reached ("low glucose suspend" feature), thereby reducing time the patient is hypoglycemic without increasing hyperglycemia. Technology is always advancing, and predictive algorithms can suspend insulin delivery to prevent as well as reduce hypoglycemia. A CGM system may be especially useful for patients who have hypoglycemia unawareness, frequent nocturnal hypoglycemia, severe hypoglycemia, or difficulty achieving target BG levels (Rubin 2011). Their use with pump therapy in children (Frontino 2012) and adolescents (Slover 2012) and during pregnancy and gestational diabetes (Combs 2012) is also beneficial.

# Basal Rate Adjustment

Do not make any basal rate changes in the first 24 h after pump start-up unless there is a blatant need, such as repeated or severe hypoglycemia or hyperglycemia. Hypoglycemia may be due to the lingering effects of prepump long-acting insulin. Also, the new pump user is commonly anxious for the first day or two; making changes in the initial basal rate or adding a second rate may be premature.

The first step in dealing with out-of-target glucose levels is to check and correct the basal rate(s). Changing the insulin-to-carbohydrate ratio or CF before correcting the basal rate(s) will not necessarily solve the problem of erratic glucose readings. The basal rate(s) is correct if the patient can skip or delay meals and 4-h postprandial readings fall within target, not varying by >30 mg/dl from the premeal glucose level. Explain the goal of establishing appropriate basal rates to the patient this way: "If you were to fast for 24 h and did not have or do anything to affect your glucose level, such as food, exercise, stress, illness, or hormonal changes, your basal rates should not let your glucose readings vary by more than 30 mg/dl throughout the entire 24 h." The 3:00 a.m. and fasting blood glucose readings should be within 30 mg/dl of the previous day's bedtime glucose reading. This is the goal when checking basal rates.

To check basal rates, first fix the fasting glucose. Remember that the patient spends approximately one-third of a 24-h day sleeping, i.e., blood glucose is not affected by bolus insulin doses during this time. A bedtime BG value within target range followed by an elevated or decreased fasting blood glucose (FBG) value approximately 8 hours later indicates the need to change the overnight basal rate. Ask the patient to:

1. Check and record the bedtime glucose reading. Do not correct it. If the bedtime glucose has been consistently <70 mg/dl or >240 mg/dl, decrease or increase the pre-evening meal bolus before performing the basal rate check again. The patient should always treat for hypoglycemia.
2. Check and record the 3:00 a.m. glucose reading. If hypoglycemic (<70 mg/dl [ADA 2013]), treat. You may need to decrease the basal rate that covers bedtime to 3:00 a.m. Do not correct for a 3:00 a.m. hyperglycemic reading unless the patient is symptomatic or has a glucose reading >240 mg/dl.
3. Check and record the fasting glucose level.
4. Compare the three readings. Increase or decrease the basal rate by 10–20% (may be 0.05 or 0.10) beginning at the time of the last glucose check preceding the glucose elevation.

*Example*
- Basal rate is 0.8 units/h × 24 h.
- 4-h postprandial bedtime glucose at 11:00 p.m. is 186 mg/dl.
- 3:00 a.m. glucose is 202 mg/dl.

**Solution:** There are two possibilities. If the 7:45 a.m. fasting glucose is 248 mg/dl, the patient has a strong dawn phenomenon. A second and higher basal rate needs to be initiated at 3:00 a.m. to correct the elevated fasting glucose reading. Increase the 0.8 units/h rate to 0.9 units/h for the period from 3:00 to 8:00 a.m., and repeat the basal check test the next evening. Repeat and increase by 0.1-unit increments until the fasting glucose is within 30 mg/dl of the 3:00 a.m. reading. However, if the 7:45 a.m. fasting glucose is 197 mg/dl, a different basal rate from 11:00 p.m. to 8:00 a.m. is not needed because all three glucose readings are within the same range. Instead, the elevated bedtime glucose reading needs to be corrected. Either the early evening-to-bedtime basal rate needs to be increased or the insulin-to-carbohydrate ratio for the evening meal needs to be increased. Once the fasting glucose is "fixed," additional basal rate checks may be needed to correct erratic daytime-to-bedtime glucose readings.

Basal rate checks require fasting and are best done in blocks of time versus a 24-h fast. Identify the postprandial period that requires alteration and choose the block of time to check, i.e., breakfast to lunch, lunch to dinner, or dinner to bedtime. To perform a basal rate check, ask the patient to choose a day free of influence of exercise, stress, menstrual hormone surges, etc.

1. Check and record a 2- to 4-h PPG level (premeal bolus given normally). Do not correct unless hypoglycemic.
2. Check and record glucose every 1–2 h for the next 4–6 h, or however long the patient is willing to fast.
3. Compare the results. If glucose has risen or fallen >30 mg/dl from the previous reading, the basal rate needs to be changed.
4. Implement a basal rate change in 0.025-, 0.05-, or 0.1-unit increments (10–20%) beginning at the time preceding the last glucose rise or fall.

*Example*
- 7:00 a.m. to 4:00 p.m. basal rate is 0.6 units/h.
- FBG is 108 mg/dl, within target. Breakfast is at 7:00 a.m.
- 3-h breakfast (10:00 a.m.) PPG: 123 mg/dl.
- 4-h breakfast (11:00 a.m.) PPG: 119 mg/dl.
- Omit lunch.
- 5-h breakfast (12:00 p.m.) PPG: 148 mg/dl.
- 6-h breakfast (1:00 p.m.) PPG: 192 mg/dl.

**Solution:** An increase in the basal rate is needed starting at 11:00 a.m., which is 1 h before the first glucose elevation begins. Increase the basal rate to 0.7 units/h from 11:00 a.m. to 3:00 p.m. Ask the patient to perform another basal rate check a few days later beginning with lunch, i.e., the patient should eat lunch (with premeal bolus taken as normal) then check glucose hourly for 5–6 h afterward. Make adjustments in 0.025-, 0.05-, or 0.1-unit increments as needed. The patient may need to perform basal rate checks over several days to determine appropriate 24-h rates.

For patients whose initial or corrected basal rates are >1.0 units/h, an increase or decrease in increments >0.1 unit may be indicated. A basal rate change should be between 10 and 20%. Be conservative.

**It is essential that the basal rates are correct.** Repeated adjustments of the insulin-to-carb ratio(s) and correction factor(s) without confirming the basal rate(s) may lead to frustration and resultant unexplainable hypo- and hyperglycemia. As stated previously, correct basal rates will maintain the pump user's SMBG values within a 30 mg/dl range throughout a 24-h period (assuming there are no other factors that affect BG values, such as exercise, stress, alcohol, menses, etc.).

# Additional Basal Rates and Establishing Basal Patterns

Pumps provide flexibility for mealtimes and fine-tuning insulin doses. The background, or basal rate of insulin, can be set for different amounts at different times of the day, depending on the user's individual needs. Today's pumps can be set for different 24-hour basal rate programs.

Basal rate requirements can differ day-to-day, depending on hormonal changes (e.g., stage of menstrual cycle for menstruating women), physical activity, and work schedules. Ideally, when basal rates are properly set, blood glucose levels do not fluctuate by more than 30 mg/dl.

Basal rates that are correctly set permit the pump user to delay or skip meals, have more flexibility with meal choices, and sleep later than their usual wake-up time. Basal rates must be set correctly to determine the correct insulin-to-carbohydrate ratio.

Insulin pumps have the option to set several different 24-h basal patterns as well as a temporary basal rate, depending on the user's personal

Remember, all pump clocks begin at midnight, so even if a basal rate is the same from 6:00 p.m. to 3:00 a.m., there will be two basal rates programmed in the pump: a 6:00 p.m. to 12:00 a.m. rate, and a 12:00 a.m. to 3:00 a.m. rate.

Examples of alternate basal rates (in units per hour) for one patient:
Weekday pattern (limited physical activity)
12 a.m.–3 a.m.: 0.5
3 a.m.–8 a.m.: 0.7
8 a.m.–5 p.m.: 0.6
5 p.m.–12 a.m.: 0.5

Weekend pattern (increased physical activity for two days)
12 a.m.–3 a.m.: 0.35
3 a.m.–8 a.m.: 0.55
8 a.m.–5 p.m.: 0.45
5 p.m.–12 a.m.: 0.35

needs. As the pump wearer progresses in learning how to identify glucose patterns or trends, such as an extended duration of hypoglycemia following exercise, or several days of hyperglycemia before the onset of menses, temporary basal rates lasting several hours to a few days and alternate 24-h basal patterns can be established. Basal rate changes are best made gradually in small increments, such as 0.05 or 0.1 units/hour, or 10% and entail additional SMBG, record keeping, and trial-and-error. Additionally, as this information is learned over time, the pump user may need refresher training from the pump manufacturer's user manual or pump trainer in the "buttonology" or "how to press the buttons to set a temporary basal rate or set up a new basal pattern."

# Temporary Basal Rates

A temporary (temp) basal rate is programmed in percentages of the usual or chosen basal pattern. Options vary depending on the brand of pump. A typical range of a temporary basal rate can be from 0 to 200% of the usual basal rate, programmable in 10% increments for up to 24 hours. Using a temp basal rate during or after exercise can help prevent hypoglycemia. For example, after swimming, a pumper can program their pump to deliver a temp rate of 80% for the next 4 hours. This equates to a 20% reduction in the pumper's basal rate(s) for the 4 hours following completion of the increased physical activity when hypoglycemia might be likely to occur. Refer to "Exercise and Physical Activity", page 122 for additional information.

Another example of using a temp rate is a pre-menses female patient who programs a temp rate higher than her usual rate to account for hormonal surges that cause hyperglycemia. Based on experience, she can program her pump to deliver 130% of her usual basal rate(s) for 24 hours. This increase is 30% higher than her "usual" basal rate.

After a programmed temporary rate has been delivered, the pump resets itself to the user's "usual" basal rate(s). Pumps offer the option of an alert/alarm reminder during and/or at the conclusion of a temp basal rate setting.

Remind the patient that using temporary basal rates and alternate basal patterns are considered advanced pump therapy options to help achieve and maintain improved glycemic control.

Pumps offer the user options to program temporary basal rate changes as well as several 24-hour basal patterns. Examples of the need for a temporary basal rate (increased or decreased) and/or alternate basal pattern (see Chapter 7 for additional information), include:

- exercise (ranging from a few hours preceding during, and several or many hours following, depending on the intensity)
- intimacy/sexual activity (ranging from a few to several hours preceding, during, and following, depending on the circumstances)
- illness (sickness, surgery)
- pre-menses (hormonal surges)
- stress (including personal, work, school)
- travel (sitting for long periods of time, changing time zones)
- vacation (less or more activity than usual)
- weekend (different exercise levels, sleep hours, amount of stress)

Example of a temporary basal rate for stress using the weekday pattern:

12 a.m.−3 a.m.: 0.5

3 a.m.−8 a.m.: 0.7

8 a.m.−5 p.m.: 0.6

2 p.m.−4 p.m.: Temporary basal increase of 30% for job-related stress: 0.6 × 130% for 2 hours = basal rate of 0.78 u/hour for this time period. The pump automatically configures the correct rate based on user's programming of +30% and automatically resumes the preset basal rate of 0.6 u/hour at 4 p.m. for continuation to 5 p.m.

5 p.m.−12 a.m.: 0.5

# Insulin-to-Carbohydrate Ratio Adjustment

After the 24-h basal rates have been determined, the patient should continue to monitor and record intake, glucose, bolus doses, exercise, etc., for your review. If PPG readings are not within target, the insulin-to-carbohydrate ratio needs adjusting. This is common and takes time to correct.

## Postprandial Hyperglycemia

Postprandial hyperglycemia requires more insulin to cover (less) carbohydrate. To correct postprandial hyperglycemia, **increase** the insulin-to-carbohydrate ratio by 3–5 grams carbohydrate.

*Example*
- Basal rates have been determined by basal check tests.
- Insulin-to-carbohydrate ratio is 1 unit:15 g. The patient counted carbohydrate and calculated the meal bolus accurately and correctly.
- 3-h PPG is 210 mg/dl.

**Solution:** Increase the insulin-to-carbohydrate ratio to 1:12, continue monitoring, and increase the ratio as needed.

## Postprandial Hypoglycemia

Postprandial hypoglycemia requires less insulin to cover (more) carbohydrate. To correct postprandial hypoglycemia, **decrease** the insulin-to-carbohydrate ratio by 3–5 grams.

*Example*
- Basal rates have been determined by basal check tests.
- Insulin-to-carbohydrate ratio is 1 unit:15 g. The patient counted carbohydrate and calculated meal bolus accurately and correctly.
- 3-h PPG is 72 mg/dl.

**Solution:** Decrease the insulin-to-carbohydrate ratio to 1:20, continue monitoring, and decrease the ratio as needed.

Sometimes patients require different ratios for different meals. An insulin pump option allows a patient to input different ICRs based on time of day. Another consideration in reviewing the insulin-to-carbohydrate ratio and meal bolus is to spread the bolus out over several hours, i.e., use an extended or "square wave" bolus. Spreading the bolus out over several hours may help prevent unexplained or troublesome postprandial hypoglycemia or hyperglycemia. Using an extended/square wave bolus or a combination partial standard (immediate)-delivery with a partial extended-delivery ("dual wave") bolus when eating pizza, high-protein, high-fat, or high-fiber foods/meals is a common practice to help correct the early postprandial hypoglycemia and a several-hour delayed hyperglycemic reading (Heinemann 2009). An extended or combination bolus is also helpful for the patient who uses pramlintide (Armstrong 2008, King 2009), or who has delayed gastric emptying or gastroparesis (see Chapter 5, "Pump Start-Up", and Chapter 7, "Other Considerations in Pump Therapy Management").

# Correction (Sensitivity) Factor Adjustment

After the 24-h basal rates have been established and the ICR ratio(s) are determined, if the patient continues to experience postprandial hyperglycemia, the correction (sensitivity) factor (CF) may need to be adjusted. Note that insulin pumps have a default "insulin on board" setting of ~3–4 hours. When the patient inputs his/her blood glucose value for a correction bolus, the pump automatically calculates the amount of active insulin from the most recent correction, meal, or total bolus ("insulin on board," depending on the pump model and features) and will provide a suggested, and in some cases, reduced correction bolus. The patient can choose to deliver the recommended reduced bolus, or may choose to override it. Caution the patient that delivering too much of a correction bolus of insulin in too short a time (while the most recent bolus is still active, "stacking" insulin) can result in postprandial hypoglycemia.

A correctly calculated CF bolus allows an elevated postprandial blood glucose level to return to target within ~3–4 h with rapid-acting insulin (the decrease takes about 5 h with short-acting insulin, which is rarely used in today's pumps). The patient should track the glucose level hourly for several hours after a correction bolus to determine the effectiveness of the CF.

If the 3- to 4-h post-bolus glucose level is still elevated, the CF needs to be increased.

*Example*
- John's 3-h PPG is 276 mg/dl. He realizes the premeal insulin bolus was too small for his meal and his pump calculates a correction bolus according to his target and CF.
- John's 3- to 4-h PPG target is 100 mg/dl and his CF is 50 mg/dl.
- 276 – 100 = 176 mg/dl above target.
- 176 mg/dl ÷ 50 mg/dl = 3.52, so John's pump calculates the correction bolus to be 3.5 units.
- John rechecks his glucose 3 h after the 3.5-unit bolus, and his glucose is 165 mg/dl, 65 mg/dl above his target. His CF needs to be changed.
- Instead of using 1 unit to lower glucose by 50 mg/dl, John tries a new CF of 40 mg/dl, i.e., 1 unit lowers his glucose 40 mg/dl.

Patients may need to try different CFs before the correct CF is identified. Caution patients not to "overlap" or "stack" bolus doses, i.e., administer a correction bolus no sooner than 3 h after a rapid-acting insulin meal bolus (and no sooner than 5 h after a short-acting insulin meal bolus). The practice of delivering too many correction boluses within a short period of time is often referred to as "stacking" insulin. The 1700 or 1500 Rule may be applicable and may need to be recalculated if the patient's pump TDD has changed. (For CF calculations, see Chapter 5.)

# Infusion Site and Tubing Concerns

Refer to "Infusion Set Insertion" in Chapter 4 for guidance on choosing and preparing an infusion site and infusion set base insertion. In general, advise the insulin pumper to check their site (and tubing, if applicable) every few hours for signs of dislodgement, redness, bumps, leakage, and air gaps in the tubing (if applicable).

## Keeping the Set Base/Pod Attached

Patients who have profuse sweating, a great amount of body hair, or engage in water-exposure sports for extended periods of time may sometimes experience problems with adherence of the set base/pod. Using a bio-occlusive skin preparation product (such as a wipe or dressing) before insertion may help with adherence as well as prevent infection. Products to help with adhesion include: Applicate's Compound Benzoin Swabstick, Drysol, Mastisol, and Skin Tach H. Pump manufacturers can provide a list of available products. An odorless antiperspirant (not deodorant) applied directly to the skin can also be beneficial. For those with excessive body hair, shaving the site in advance will help with dressing/tape adherence. Some patients may prefer the "sandwich" method, using two dressings: prepare the skin, apply a dressing first, then insert the set base, and then place additional tape or dressing over the base. Cutting a hole in the second dressing will allow the tubing to be easily disconnected. Another option is use just one additional dressing, cut a hole in it to allow the tubing to be disconnected, and place it over the inserted base. Advise the pump patient to make sure the skin is completely dry before applying the set base/pod. "Stretching" the skin before applying the set (or dressing/tape) will aid in comfort, and prevent the skin from feeling "pinched" below the tape.

After insertion, additional sterile dressing or tape may help anchor the set base and prevent accidental dislodgement. Making a "safety loop" with a few inches of the tubing and using additional dressing or tape to anchor the loop can help with adhesion. Commercial products include: Durapore, Micropore, Transpore and other silk- or silk-like tape and IV 3000™, Bioclusive, Polyskin II, and Tegaderm dressing. The additional tape or dressing can be especially useful during exercise, water sports, and intimacy. Some people find that making a safety loop and/or using "extra" tape or dressing is a way to prevent accidental dislodgment during daily routine activities, such as using the bathroom and changing clothes.

## Site Rotation

A very important general recommendation for the new pumper is to rotate their infusion site and change their infusion set base/pod every two to three days. An infusion set "base" (the part of the infusion set that is attached to the skin) or pod remains in place for several days with self-adhesive tape. Over time and with experience of having left a set base/pod unchanged for too many days, patients will learn the optimal duration of time between set changes and site rotation. If the set base/pod and site remain unchanged too long, for example, over three days, various problems can result, including: redness, irritation, tenderness or soreness at the site, scarring below the skin, lipohypertrophy, and hyperglycemia (from poor insulin absorption). The pump patient who does not rotate their site as recommended also increases their risk of repeated infections. Caution your patients that it is crucial to change the infusion site/set at an established duration of time. Currently, pump patients must develop their own record-keeping method to be reminded to change their sites routinely. A "site change reminder" alarm/alert pump feature is an ideal way for the patient to be reminded to rotate and change their site and set/pod. As of this writing, newer smart pumps do not offer this feature, but this would be an excellent alarm/alert for convenience as well as necessity.

Infusion sites should be rotated so that the next site is at least 2 to 3 inches from the previous site. The navel/belly-button area should be avoided, as the skin is tender. Using a pattern of a "clock" (curve), a horizontal or vertical "M" or "W," a criss-cross, or a zigzag and rotating from side to side helps the pumper to keep track of site rotation. When changing infusion sites from one area of the body to another (for example, abdomen to thigh), advise the patient to check their blood glucose more frequently, as insulin absorption differs from area to area.

The best time to rotate the infusion site and change the set base/pod and is when the skin is clean and dry, such as immediately after a shower or bath (exfoliated skin can aid in adhesion), or preceding a meal. Additionally, a site/set change should occur when there's at least four hours of time available afterwards to check blood glucose. This helps to confirm the infusion set base or pod is properly in place and the site is a "good" site, i.e., free of scar tissue or lipohypertrophy. When a set base/pod is changed just before sleep and there's a problem with improper insertion, hitting scar tissue, kinking, or leakage, hyperglycemia can result.

**Sets with tubing: change the set base but not the insulin cartridge/reservoir and/or the tubing?**

Many experienced pumpers change their set base as recommended, but choose not to change the tubing that attaches to the base until the insulin in the cartridge/reservoir is depleted. This can save time and insulin usage and aids in convenience. Since the insulin is constantly being infused through the tubing, and the cartridge or reservoir holds more than a typical three-day amount of insulin (180 to 310 units), discarding the tubing and changing the more-than-three-day-supply-of-insulin cartridge/reservoir every two to three days can be wasteful and takes a few extra minutes of time. Remember that the tubing contains insulin that is discarded every time the tubing is changed.

HOWEVER, the pumper must consider the safety and efficacy of the insulin remaining in the cartridge/reservoir that is at body temperature and/or exposed to temperature changes over the course of several days, i.e., days beyond the two to three recommended for a site change. Decades ago, an insulin pump manufacturer offered an infusion set with two bases and one set of tubing, and this particular set was a popular option. Apidra is approved for use in a pump cartridge/reservoir for up to 48 hours (sanofi-aventis 2009); Humalog, up to six days in the cartridge/reservoir and up to three in the tubing (Eli Lilly 2011); and NovoLog, up to six-day usage in an insulin pump (Novo Nordisk 2002–2011). The practice of rotating the site and changing the set base but not the tubing warrants careful consideration. The pumper who chooses to "experiment" with this practice must carefully consider the repercussions, such as gradual increases in blood glucose due to the possible decreasing efficacy of the insulin. Some experienced pumpers fill their cartridge/reservoir with enough insulin for two set base changes, while others who are more insulin sensitive (thus use less insulin) have tried three or four set base changes before changing the tubing, waiting until their cartridge/reservoir is depleted. Exercise caution, including awareness of unexplained gradual blood glucose increases, for your patient who considers this option.

## Site Irritation and Set/Pod Removal

Some people may experience irritation, such as itching or tenderness, at the site. Site irritation can be from the dressing/tape adhesive or keeping the set/pod in place too long. Sensitivity or allergy to a particular component in the adhesive or the dressing/tape is uncommon but can happen. Patients who seem to be more prone to infection may be colonized with staphlococcus aureus. Such patients may benefit from enhanced site cleaning with a product designed to kill staphlococcus, such as Hibiclens.

Some pumpers experience a rash while the dressing/tape is in place or after removing the set/pod. Residual adhesive may be a cause of irritation at the site after the set base/pod is removed. Using a bio-occlusive skin preparation product (such as a wipe or dressing) before insertion may help to separate the irritant from the skin (Kaufman 2012) and thorough cleansing of the skin after a set removal can help prevent site irritation. Use of a commercial product, such as Benzoin, Detachol, or Uni-Solve may help remove excess adhesive.

## "Pump Bumps"

A small asymptomatic hematoma, or "pump bump," is the body's normal reaction to a foreign object and usually occurs when a set base or pod has been in place too long. These hematomas disappear over time, and patients should avoid insertion close to a hematoma. If the patient notices a gradual or unexplained increase in blood glucose, changing the site and set/pod (as the first step to returning the blood glucose to target) is advised. "When in doubt, change it out" is a common mantra for experienced pumpers. Examine a pumper's infusion sites at every routine visit.

## Insulin Leakage

Occasionally, the pump patient may experience insulin tubing leakage that can be caused by a number of factors, including: loose connection at the hub/Luer lock; loose connection to the set base; broken tubing; or, though rare, kinked tubing. If any of these events occur, the pump may not sound an alarm, as the insulin will continue to be infused out of the cartridge/tubing and the pump may not detect an interruption or cessation of the infusion after the insulin travels through the hub. Remind the patient that insulin has an odor similar to a wet bandage. If the patient experiences unexplained hyperglycemia, the connection of the set base/pod to the body as well as the connection of the tubing to the base or pump cartridge/reservoir and the tubing itself should be considered. Retightening the tubing may solve the problem, but if there is too much of a gap between the tubing and the hub of the pump cartridge/reservoir, changing the tubing altogether is advised, as retightening the tubing may create air bubbles or gaps.

## Air Bubbles in the Tubing

Occasionally, air bubbles or air "space" may appear in the tubing. Air bubbles are very tiny and are often described as the size of champagne bubbles. Air space appears as an opaque "gap" in the insulin in the tubing and can be from a fraction of an inch to several inches in length. Causes of tiny bubbles or air gaps include: (1) filling the cartridge/reservoir with cold insulin—as the insulin comes to room temperature, it expands and can create air spaces in the tubing; (2) air that was contained within the insulin vial prior to filling the cartridge/reservoir—a vial that has been shaken may contain air bubbles; (3) disconnecting and reconnecting the tubing at the Luer lock (cartridge/reservoir) connection—the air space at the hub end of the tubing loses the insulin when disconnected, and after reconnection, the space fills prior to the tubing, and air bubbles/gaps form and travel through the tubing.

Large amounts of air (1/4 inch) in the tubing will result in a decreased amount of insulin infusion, either basal, bolus, or both. One inch of tubing contains approximately 0.3 to 0.5 unit of insulin (varies depending on the brand of infusion set). Advise the pumper to check their tubing every few hours and to be on the lookout for air gaps.

To remove the air in the tubing, advise the pumper to

(a) disconnect the tubing at the base (NOT at the cartridge/reservoir connection) end.

(b) hold the tubing in mid-air and deliver either a primed amount of insulin (using the "prime" function) or a bolus.

(c) watch the insulin and air travel through the tubing.

(d) when insulin is dripping from the tubing end and there are no more visible air bubbles or gaps, stop the process.

(e) reconnect the tubing to the base. Patients should continue to monitor their blood glucose and take action accordingly.

## Blood in the Tubing

Blood in the tubing results from blood at the subcutaneous site that has "backed up," traveled through the cannula or needle, and entered the tubing. This may or may not cause an occlusion and/or malabsorption of the insulin. An occlusion can occur when the cannula or needle has been inserted into scar tissue. Depending on the severity of the occlusion and sensitivity of the pump occlusion detection system, an occlusion alarm can occur, alerting the pump user to take action. In tubeless pumps, blood may not be visible, but the pump nonetheless has detected an occlusion and alerted the pumper. Advise the patient to never continue the insulin infusion or deliver a bolus to push the blood back through the tubing. To take action, the pump user should remove both the set and tubing (or pod), and complete a new "set up," including a site change, preferably several inches from the previous site), set/pod change, and tubing change (if applicable). Monitoring the blood glucose closely for several hours is important.

## Infections

The metal/steel needle or Teflon cannula is a foreign body inserted subcutaneously, thus, infection can result, especially if bacteria were introduced at the time of insertion or when the set remains in place for an extended period of time. If the pumper breathes or sneezes on or touches the metal/steel needle or cannula before insertion, bacteria can also be introduced subcutaneously. Before insertion and after cleansing the infusion site, applying a bio-occlusive adhesive dressing (see "Infusion Set Insertion" in Chapter 4) to the skin can help protect the site from additional bacteria at the point of insertion.

Advise the pump patient to be aware of signs of a site infection, such as discomfort, inflammation or redness, pain, swelling, tenderness, and warmth. Remind the pump patient that people with diabetes are more likely than others to be carriers of staph (staphylococcus), and thus, are at greater risk of acquiring a site infection. Encourage the patient to notify their HCP if he/she suspects an infection, as immediate medical attention can prevent further problems.

# Emergency Supplies

Prepare your patients to deal with the worst possible situation. Caution the new pump patient to always be prepared for problems, such as an infusion set that becomes dislodged or "falls off," leaky or broken tubing, running out of insulin (ignoring the pump's alerts that the volume of insulin is low), dead battery in the pump or remote control, or, worst-case scenario, a pump remote or pump PDA failure, or theft because it was mistaken for a cell phone or MP3 player.

Pumps have fallen off while the patient was closing the car door, leaving the infusion set attached to the body but cut by the car door, with the pump left on the road. Pets (notably cats and dogs) may disconnect or chew through an infusion set without the user's awareness or knowledge—especially during nocturnal or sleep hours. Physical activity, excessive perspiration, unplanned exposure to water, and even clothes shopping can dislodge or cause accidental removal of the infusion set. A dropped pump can break. And a static electrical discharge from the pump wearer or a pet can disrupt the electrical circuitry of the pump. A malfunctioning pump, a pump remote or pump PDA failure or theft, or even a severe infusion site infection constitutes an emergency.

People who wear insulin pumps must be prepared at all times with a back up system to continue insulin delivery. Pump patients no longer have intermediate- or long-acting insulin in their body to protect them from the rapid onset of ketosis or ketoacidosis.

Access to a rapid-acting insulin analog pen and pen needles or vial and syringes is essential. Injecting a rapid-acting analog every 3 to 4 hours can hold the person over until s/he can obtain a basal insulin.

All people with diabetes should wear some form of medical identification. A pump patient's medical identification should indicate "on insulin pump" or "uses insulin pump."

A back up plan includes:

- Insulin dosage guidelines for being "off the pump," including recommendations for basal insulin (prescription and dose[s]) and bolus insulin (prescription and dose[s])
- (Include a prescription for pen needles or insulin syringes, whichever is preferred by the patient)
- Contact information: who the patient should contact for medical/clinical assistance (you, as their HCP) and who should be contacted for technical pump issues, such as forgetting how to program the pump, or assistance for a pump malfunction or failure (pump trainer or manufacturer)

A well-trained pump patient should know the basic "button push-ing" operations of their pump, including how to: view their basal rates/pattern, change or set basal rates, implement alternate basal patterns, set a temp basal rate, implement bolus options, such as an extended/square wave and combination/dual wave bolus, view history (last bolus[es], TDD, BG values), etc. (see Chapter 7, Other Considerations in Pump Therapy Management). If the pump patient does not know how to operate their pump, your recommendations for changes cannot be implemented. If you notice a pattern of patients who have been trained by a manufacturer's pump trainer(s) but lack basic pump operation knowledge, contact the pump trainer(s) to take corrective action.

Advise the new pumper to always have spare items readily available and within arm's reach, such as in a purse, backpack, briefcase, car console/glove compartment, etc. Back up supplies are essential and include:

- Treatment for hypoglycemia
- Glucose meter, lancets, meter batteries, and strips
- Infusion set(s) or pod(s) (two recommended)
- Pump cartridge/reservoir
- Pump software components, including pre-filled insulin cartridge, if applicable
- Skin prep pad or other site preparation supplies
- Alcohol swab (or other cleansing agent)
- Site dressing or tape (if used)
- Rapid-acting insulin analog vial for syringe use or to fill pump cartridge/reservoir (remind the patient about insulin expiration date and storage)
- Syringe(s) for injections (for use with vial)
- Rapid-acting insulin analog pen and pen needles (if not carrying rapid-acting insulin analog vial and syringe [remind the patient about insulin expiration date and storage])
- Pump battery, charger, and insertion/removal tools, if necessary
- Physician name, address, and phone numbers
- Emergency contact addresses and phone numbers

Additional helpful items include a vial or pen of long-acting insulin to replace the pump's basal rate(s) and dosage guidelines for the patient. Ketone test strips— for blood if the patient uses a glucose meter that can also check for ketones—or urine ketone test strips are also recommended. Treatment for hypoglycemia that does not have a perishable expiration date or require refrigeration, such as glucose tablets, glucose gel, soft chewable non-chocolate or melting candy, and cake icing in tubes, is essential. The patient should also consider the availability of glucagon (which requires a prescription and teaching the patient's significant other or support personnel) for at-home emergency as well as outside-home (office, work site, etc.) use.

# Troubleshooting

A summary of specific troubleshooting adjustment options appear below in Tables 4 and 5.

| TABLE 4. Possible Causes of Hyperglycemia and Adjustment Options | |
|---|---|
| **Possible Cause** | **Adjustment Options** |
| Insufficient insulin to cover carbohydrate | Inaccurate carbohydrate counting (e.g., misjudgment of portion size(s), omitting carb content of mixers in alcoholic beverages, breading on meat, poultry, fish, etc.); review carbohydrate calculations. The insulin-to-carbohydrate ratio (ICR) may be too low; consider increasing. Example: use 1 unit of insulin to cover less carbohydrate, e.g., 1 unit for 12 g instead of 1 unit for 15 g. Bolus may have been missed. Set missed meal bolus alerts/alarms to prevent omission of bolus dose(s). |
| Excessive intake of protein and/or fat | Consider splitting the bolus dose— use extended (square wave) or combination (dual wave) bolus feature OR set an increased temporary basal rate(s). |

*(Table continues on next page)*

**TABLE 4. Possible Causes of Hyperglycemia and Adjustment Options** *(Continued)*

| Possible Cause | Adjustment Options |
| --- | --- |
| Insufficient basal insulin | Basal rate(s) are inaccurate. Perform basal rate tests. |
| Insulin timing not matched to meal intake | Review timing of bolus(es). |
| Insulin dose not timed to account for delayed digestion due to gastroparesis or use of pramlintide | For gastroparesis: discuss potential use of GI motility medications.<br>For pramlintide: review timing and effects of pramlintide.<br>Consider use of extended (square wave) or combination (dual wave) bolus.<br>Consider use of extended or combination bolus feature OR decreased/increased temporary basal rate(s). |
| Bolus insulin dose omitted | Set pump alarm or alert reminder for missed bolus and/or high blood glucose. |
| Inaccurate Correction/Sensitivity Factor (CF/SF) | Use lower CF. Example: 1 unit of insulin lowers glucose 40 mg/dl instead of 50 mg/dl. |
| Too much time between correction bolus doses | Review duration of insulin action time.<br>Decrease time between bolus correction doses.<br>Adjust and follow insulin-on-board/duration of insulin action settings and reminders. |
| Overtreatment of hypoglycemia | Review "Rule of 15": consume 15 grams of carbohydrate and check blood glucose in 15 minutes; if not at target, repeat treatment until blood glucose reaches target.<br>Review appropriate treatment for hypoglycemia: type and amount of carbohydrate.<br>Use correction bolus feature (for reverse recommendation). |

## TABLE 4. Possible Causes of Hyperglycemia and Adjustment Options *(Continued)*

| Possible Cause | Adjustment Options |
| --- | --- |
| Decrease in usual exercise or physical activity | Increase ICR(s). Example: use 1 unit of insulin to cover less carbohydrate, e.g., 1:12 instead of 1:15. Decrease CF(s). Example: 1 unit of insulin lowers blood glucose 40 mg/dl instead of 50 mg/dl. |
| Initiation of new medication or dosage change | Consider changing basal rate(s); increase basal rate(s) on days with less exercise; implement temporary increased basal rate for several hours or alternate non-exercise day basal profile. Review and confirm correct dose(s). Review blood glucose effects of new medications, e.g., addition of glucocorticoid. |
| Onset of illness; dental surgery; other surgeries | Notify healthcare professional. Increase basal rate(s), ICR(s), and decrease CF(s) as needed. Notify healthcare professional. Check ketones (especially with type 1 diabetes). Increase non-caloric fluids if appropriate. Increase diabetes medication doses. Implement increased temporary basal rates. Increase ICR(s) and decrease CF(s), if needed. |
| Emotional stress | Review intake: eating more than usual? Increase basal rate(s); consider use of temporary increased basal rate(s). Increase ICR(s) and decrease CF(s). |
| Menses/hormonal changes | Consider alternate higher basal rates or temporary increased basal rates. Increase ICR(s) and decrease CF(s). |

*(Table continues on next page)*

## TABLE 4. Possible Causes of Hyperglycemia and Adjustment Options

| Possible Cause | Adjustment Options |
| --- | --- |
| May be using incorrect basal rates (24-hour or temporary), target glucose level(s), ICR(s), CF(s), or duration of insulin action/on-board insulin settings | Review pump time/date selection, basal rate selection/programming (24-hour or temporary), target glucose level(s), ICR(s), CF(s), and duration-of-insulin-action (on-board insulin) settings. If incorrect, reprogram. |
| Battery(ies) may be dead; alarm ignored or not heard/felt | Replace or charge battery(ies). |
| Insulin cartridge/reservoir empty | Replace cartridge/reservoir. |
| Insulin may have deteriorated. | Verify insulin has not expired. |
| Tubing or pod may be occluded, contain air, have become dislodged or broken, or have cracks | Replace tubing/infusion set or pod. |
| Infusion site red, irritated due to infection, or set not changed within two to three days or according to schedule | Change site and set more frequently. Set a pump site/set change reminder alarm. |

**Notes:**
It's best to fine-tune insulin doses related to carbohydrate first before making other insulin dose changes.
Always try one method at a time.
Planned exercise does not guarantee a decrease in hyperglycemia. People with diabetes may experience hyperglycemia if they exercise while under-insulinized or with the presence of ketones. Refer to "Exercise and Physical Activity" in Chapter 7.
To correct preprandial hyperglycemia, people can be encouraged to take one or more immediate actions:
1. Increase the amount of the preprandial insulin dose, based on the CF.
2. Decrease the amount of carbohydrate at the meal, but do not increase the preprandial insulin bolus dose. Base the amount of reduced carbohydrate on the CF—the person should know the amount of carbohydrate that will increase their blood glucose a certain number of mg/dl and then deduct the carbohydrate amount accordingly.
3. Use the pump setting that suggests an increased amount of insulin, i.e., an individualized appropriate correction dose based on the programmed CF and target glucose level.

## TABLE 5.  Possible Causes of Hypoglycemia and Adjustment Options

| Possible Cause | Adjustment Options |
| --- | --- |
| Too much insulin to cover carbohydrate | Inaccurate carbohydrate counting; review carbo-hydrate calculations.<br>The ICR may be too high; decrease. Example: use 1 unit of insulin to cover more carbohydrate, e.g., 1:15 instead of 1:12. |
| Decreased intake of protein and/or fat | Decrease dose(s) of basal rate(s).<br>If splitting bolus dose, reduce percentage of upfront bolus and increase percentage of remainder dose.<br>Recalculate duration of time and/or percentage of immediate and extended (square wave) or combination (dual wave) bolus durations. |
| Too much basal insulin | Decrease basal rate(s). |
| Insulin timing not matched to meal intake | Review timing of insulin dose. |
| Pramlintide dose not timed to meal intake | Review timing of pramlintide.<br>Delay meal bolus until during or after meal.<br>Use extended (square wave) or combination (dual wave) feature. |
| Insulin dose not timed to account for delayed digestion due to gastroparesis or use of pramlintide | Discuss potential use of GI motility medications.<br>Consider use of extended (square wave) or combination (dual wave) bolus OR decreased/increased temporary basal rate(s). |
| Insulin dose or diabetes medication dose unclear | Review and confirm dose(s).<br>Provide strategies to remember to take correct dose of meds, e.g., set pump reminder alarm or alert. |
| Inaccurate CF | Use higher CF. Example: 1 unit lowers more blood glucose (50 mg/dl instead of 40 mg/dl). |
| Too many correction bolus doses, i.e., "stacking insulin" | Review timing of correction bolus dose(s) and duration of insulin action.<br>Increase time between bolus correction doses.<br>Adjust and follow duration of insulin action settings and reminders. |

*(Table continues on next page)*

## TABLE 5.  Possible Causes of Hypoglycemia and Adjustment Options *(Continued)*

| Possible Cause | Adjustment Options |
|---|---|
| Increase in usual exercise or physical activity | Decrease ICR(s). Example: use 1 unit of insulin to cover more carbohydrate, e.g., 1:15 instead of 1:12.<br>Increase CF(s). Example: 1 unit of insulin lowers blood glucose 50 mg/dl instead of 40 mg/dl.<br>Consider changing basal rate(s); decrease basal rate(s) on days with less exercise.<br>Use temporary decreased basal rate for several hours or alternate nonexercise day basal profile. |
| Initiation of new medication or dosage change | Review and confirm correct dose(s).<br>Review blood glucose effects of new medications, e.g., ß-blockers. |
| Onset of illness; dental surgery; other surgeries | Notify healthcare professional.<br>Check ketones (especially with type 1 diabetes).<br>Substitute solid carbohydrate foods with liquid carbohydrate, if tolerated.<br>Possibly decrease basal rate(s) and ICR(s) and increase CF(s).<br>Consider alternate lower basal rates or temporary decreased basal rates. |
| Emotional stress | Possibly decrease basal rate(s) and ICR(s) and increase CF(s).<br>Consider alternate lower basal rates or temporary decreased basal rates. |
| Menses/hormonal changes | Decrease basal insulin rate(s) and ICR(s) and increase CF(s).<br>Consider alternate lower basal rates or temporary decreased basal rates. |
| Alcohol intake | Review alcohol intake: quantity, type.<br>Remind people that alcohol can increase the risk for recovery from hypoglycemia due to the inhibition of gluconeogenesis, possibly resulting in lower blood glucose for up to 12 hours.<br>Increase frequency of SMBG the morning after alcohol consumption.<br>Consider reducing next morning bolus insulin dose(s) or increase consumption of additional carbohydrate 6–12 hours after alcohol consumption.<br>Possibly consider using temporary decreased basal rate(s). |

## TABLE 5.  Possible Causes of Hypoglycemia and Adjustment Options *(Continued)*

| Possible Cause | Adjustment Options |
|---|---|
| May be using incorrect basal rates (24-hour or temporary), target glucose level(s), ICR(s), CF(s), and duration-of-insulin-action/on-board insulin settings | Review pump time/date selection, basal rate selection/programming (24-hour or temporary), target glucose level(s), ICR(s), CF(s), and duration-of-insulin-action settings; if incorrect, reprogram. |
| May have incorrect placement of infusion site/set or pod | Check site selection and review appropriate site selection to avoid intra-muscular placement. |

**Notes:**

It's best to fine-tune insulin doses related to carbohydrate first before making other insulin dose changes.

Always try one method at a time.

To correct preprandial hypoglycemia, people can be encouraged to take one or more immediate actions:

1. Treat the hypoglycemia with an appropriate amount of carbohydrate. Base the amount of carbohydrate on the ICR. **Do not increase the preprandial bolus dose to cover the carbohydrate consumed for the treatment of the hypoglycemia.** Clinicians often use the "Rule of 15": consume 15 grams of carbohydrate, and check blood glucose. If not at target, repeat treatment until blood glucose reaches target. The caveat is that this general rule may be too much or not enough carbohydrate for some people.

2. Use the pump setting that suggests an individualized appropriate amount of carbohydrate to increase the blood glucose level. Do not increase the preprandial bolus dose.

3. Increase the amount of carbohydrate at the meal, but do not increase the preprandial insulin bolus dose. Base the amount of additional carbohydrate on the ICR, i.e., the person should know the amount of carbohydrate that will increase their blood glucose a certain number of mg/dl and consume the amount of carbohydrate that will return levels to target. This method of treating hypoglycemia is best for people who are not concerned about weight gain, since the increased amount of carbohydrate adds calories. For those who are concerned with weight gain, reducing insulin is a better choice.

4. Use the pump setting that suggests a reduced amount of insulin for the preprandial bolus, i.e., an individualized appropriate correction dose based on the programmed CF and target glucose level.

5. Delay the preprandial insulin dose until during or after the meal. This gives the food a chance to raise blood glucose. Check blood glucose 15–20 minutes after the beginning of the meal and give the meal insulin bolus dose when glucose begins to rise.

## REFERENCES

American Diabetes Association: 2013 Clinical practice recommendations. *Diabetes Care* 36 (Suppl.1):S11–S66, 2013

Armstrong D, King A, Wolfe G: A study of insulin pump-delivered bolus wave forms with pramlintide treatment. *Diabetes* 57 (Suppl.1):A566–567,2008

Bergenstal RM, Tamborlane WV, Ahmann A, Buse JB, Dailey G, Davis SN, Joyce C, Peoples T, Perkins BA, Welsh JB, Willi SM, Wood MA; STAR 3 Study Group: Effectiveness of sensor-augmented insulin-pump therapy in type 1 diabetes. *N Engl J Med* 363:311–320, 2010

Buse JB, Kudva YC, Battelino T, Davis SN, Shin J, Welsh JB: Effects of sensor-augmented pump therapy on glycemic variability in well-controlled type 1 diabetes in the STAR-3 study. *Diabetes Technol Ther* 14:644–647. Epub Apr 23, 2012

Combs CA: Continuous glucose monitoring and insulin pump therapy for diabetes in pregnancy. *J Matern Fetal Neonatal Med.* 25:2025–7, 2012

Eli Lilly and Company: *Humalog (insulin lispro injection USP [rDNA origin]) for injection Prescribing Information.* Indianapolis, IN: Eli Lilly and Company, 2011

Frontino G, Bonfanti R, Scaramuzza A, Rabbone I, Meschi F, Rigamonti A, Battaglino R, Favalli V, Bonura C, Sicignano S, Gioia E, Zuccotti GV, Cerutti F, Chiumello G: Sensor-augmented pump therapy in very young children with type 1 diabetes: an efficacy and feasibility observational study. *Diabetes Technol Ther* 14:762–764, 2012

Heinemann L: Insulin pump therapy: What is the evidence for using different types of boluses for coverage of prandial insulin requirements? *J Diabetes Sci Technol* 3:1490–1500, 2009

Kaufman FR, Westfall E: *Insulin Pumps and Continuous Glucose Monitoring: A User's Guide to Effective Diabetes Management.* Alexandria, VA: American Diabetes Association, 2012

King AB: Continuous glucose monitoring-guided insulin dosing in pump-treated patients with type 1 diabetes: a clinical guide. *J Diabetes Sci Technol* 6:191–203, 2012

King AB, Genta F, Wolf G: A modified combination wave compared to a square wave insulin bolus in pump and pramlintide treated type 1 diabetes using continuous glucose monitoring. *Diabetes* 58S (Suppl 1):A120, 452-P, 2009

Novo Nordisk A/S: *NovoLog® (insulin aspart [rDNA origin]) injection Prescribing Information.* Novo Nordisk A/S, Bagsvaerd, Denmark, 2002–2011

Raccah D, Sulmont V, Reznik Y, Guerci B, Renard E, Hanaire H, Jeandidier N, Nicolino M: Incremental value of continuous glucose monitoring when starting pump therapy in patients with poorly controlled type 1 diabetes (The Real Trend Study). *Diabetes Care* 32:2245–2250, 2009

Rigla M, Hernando E, Gomez E, Brugues E, Garcia-Saez G, Capel I, Pons B, DeLeiva A: Real-time continuous glucose monitoring together with telemedical assistance improves glycemic control and glucose stability in pump-treated patients. *Diabetes Technol Ther* 10:194–199, 2008

Roche Insulin Delivery Systems, Inc.: *ACCU-CHEK Guide to Infusion Site Management.* Fishers, IN, 2012

Rubin RR, Borgman SK, Sulik BT. Crossing the technology divide: practical strategies for transitioning patients from multiple daily insulin injections to sensor-augmented pump therapy. *Diabetes Educ* 37 (Suppl. 1):5S–18S, 2011

sanofi-aventis: *Apidra (insulin gluslisine [rDNA origin] injection) solution for injection Prescribing Information.* Bridgewater, NJ: sanofi-aventis U.S., 2009

Slover RH, Welsh JB, Criego A, Weinzimer SA, Willi SM, Wood MA, Tamborlane WV: Effectiveness of sensor-augmented pump therapy in children and adolescents with type 1 diabetes in the STAR 3 study. *Pediatr Diabetes* 13:6–11, 2012

U.S. FDA: Medical Devices/Continuous Glucose Sensors http://google2.fda.gov/search?as_sitesearch=www.fda.gov/MedicalDevices/ProductsandMedicalProcedures/DeviceApprovalsandClearances&q=continuous+glucose+sensor&client=FDAgov&site=FDAgov&lr=&proxystylesheet=FDAgov&requiredfields=-archive:Yes&output=xml_no_dtd&getfields=*&ie=UTF-8&ip=108.3.172.150&access=p&sort=date:D:L:d1&entqr=3&entqrm=0&oe=UTF-8&ud=1 (Accessed 16 March 2013)

# Other Considerations in Pump Therapy Management

O nce the initial basal rates and insulin doses have been determined, the patient and healthcare team can continue to tailor the pump therapy. Different basal rates, ICRs, and CFs to accommodate such normal events as dining out, exercise, illness, stress, travel, and the menstrual cycle can be established. Using the "insulin on board" or "active insulin" setting and the pump's bolus calculator to determine a bolus or correction dose can assist in accurate bolus dose calculations. Taking pump therapy to this next level requires additional detailed monitoring, record keeping, and trial-and-error, but is well worthwhile.

Communication and teamwork with a CDE who is familiar and experienced with insulin pump therapy may be especially helpful for the novice pumper as well as the HCP learning to implement pump therapy.

## Use of Duration of Insulin Action "Insulin on Board" or "Active Insulin" Feature

People who use a pump must know how to synchronize the amount of prandial insulin with the amount of carbohydrate they choose to eat. Several studies (Klupa 2008, Shashaj 2008, Gross 2003) have demonstrated that use of an insulin pump's bolus calculator can effectively control postprandial glucose levels. For optimal glycemic control, prandial (bolus) insulin doses are calculated based on several factors, including target blood glucose, current blood glucose, individualized ICR(s), individualized CF(s), and the amount of insulin remaining from a previous meal/snack bolus and/or correction bolus. This amount of insulin is referred to as "insulin on board" (IOB) or "active insulin" and can be used by the pump to calculate a bolus.

The currently available rapid-acting insulin analogs have an onset of 5 to 15 minutes, peak activity between 30 and 90 minutes, and duration of about 4 to 6 hours (Hirsch 2005). The IOB or "active insulin" pump setting tells the pumper the approximate amount of bolus insulin that is active and, thus, can lower the blood glucose level. Most pumps have a default setting (example: 4 hours), but allow the duration to be programmed between 3 and 6 hours. A shorter duration of IOB may be preferred for tighter control, but puts the user at risk for hypoglycemia due to potential overlap or "stacking" of insulin doses. Pump manufacturers use a variety of methods to configure the IOB or active insulin setting. Some pumps include the most recent meal bolus in the IOB/active amount while others do not. Most pumps take into account the most recent correction bolus and subtract an amount based on time duration and the pharmacokinetics or pharmacodynamics of the insulin when calculating the correction bolus. Additionally, a pump's bolus calculator may recommend a higher bolus if the current blood glucose is above target compared to a bolus dose recommended for blood glucose at target.

Pump manufacturers vary in their methods of incorporating IOB or active insulin in calculating a meal and correction bolus. Become familiar with a pump's bolus calculator feature and setting so that you can advise your pump patients accordingly. Trial and error and keeping detailed records will help you and your pump patient determine if the pump's default IOB/active insulin time needs to be adjusted. Additionally, although the pump can recommend a bolus dose based on the factors mentioned above, it cannot account for a change in physical activity (such as increased or decreased activity). A pump user must decide to accept or override the pump's suggested bolus (refer to the upcoming section, "Exercise and Physical Activity," in this chapter). In general, the duration of action for a large bolus is longer than for small doses of insulin. After delivering a correction bolus, advise patients to not administer a second correction bolus within 2 hours of the first bolus (Hirsch 2010).

Discuss the IOB/active insulin setting with your pump patient *before* the person is to be trained on the pump. The duration of insulin action has a profound influence on the use and efficacy of correction boluses. Generally, a duration of 3 to 4 hours works for most people, but *the decision to program an appropriate insulin duration setting should be based on sound clinical judgment and should not be left to the discretion of a per diem or pump manufacturer trainer on the day of pump initiation/training.*

Factors to consider in programming an insulin pump for the "duration of insulin action" feature include:

■ Person's knowledge of and experience with:
  - "how long my insulin lasts"
  - recurrent postprandial hyperglycemia or recurrent hypoglycemia
  - the "vicious cycle" of the overtreatment of hyperglycemia resulting in hypoglycemia and/or overtreatment of hypoglycemia resulting in hyperglycemia
■ HCP's knowledge of and experience with:
  - using insulin action curves in advising a person about the "wait time" to administer a correction dose of insulin
  - the person's specific insulin requirements, including previous insulin doses, sensitivity to insulin, recurrent hyper-and hypoglycemia, and, if present, knowledge of the person's episodes of the "vicious cycle" of hyperglycemia overtreatment and hypoglycemia overtreatment
  - using insulin action curves and duration of insulin on board features

# Dining Out and Special Meals: Bolus Options

**Knowledge of carbohydrate counting is essential for success with an insulin pump.** Eating meals at home and having access to carbohydrate values of foods (such as recipe "breakdowns" and nutrition labels) can aid in carb counting accuracy and the calculation of an appropriate bolus dose. In today's world, people consume, on the average, nearly five meals a week away from home. For many people these numbers are even higher and trend data predict continued growth in dollars spent away from home (National Restaurant Association

2012). Ethnic foods and meals are gaining in popularity, and are a mainstay of today's dietary intake. People are faced with the challenge of calculating or "guesstimating" nutrient composition of meals, especially carbohydrate amounts. Some restaurants provide nutrient values, while the internet and books, as well as built-in pump databases, are other sources of information to aid the pumper in calculating correct bolus doses based on carbohydrate grams.

But what about unfamiliar ethnic or holiday foods that are a "combination" of carbohydrate, protein, and fat, or foods/meals that have a high-protein, high-fat, high-fiber, or low-glycemic index (GI) content? And what about meals that last longer than usual, such as a buffet or a celebratory/holiday meal, or "grazing" (i.e., snacking over several hours)?

Patients often estimate ("guesstimate") not only carbohydrate amounts, but the amount of protein and fat they consume. "Meat or fish or poultry doesn't contain carbohydrate, so if I eat more than 3 or 4 ounces, will that affect my blood sugar?" "Fat doesn't have carbohydrate, so why it should it affect my blood sugar?" And foods that are "high in fiber" are often promoted as having a "delayed" or lowering effect on blood glucose. Postprandial excursions after consuming high-protein or high-fat meals are not well documented. Decades ago, research in patients with type 1 diabetes using basal-bolus regimens indicated that the prandial bolus insulin doses should be based on the carbohydrate content of the meal and that the fiber, fat, and GI content did not affect the prandial insulin requirements. In that particular study, protein and fat content were constant, so the insulin needed for their metabolism was likely derived from basal insulin (Rabasa-Lhoret 1999). Anecdotally and with data from downloaded meters and CGM, meals with larger amounts of protein and fat are often reported to produce elevated postprandial glucose levels for several hours. This suggests that additional protein and fat may delay the absorption of glucose or additional prandial insulin may be necessary to cover it (Pankowska 2010). Although there exists little scientific data to support the delayed elevation of prandial glucose from protein and/or fat intake (ADA 2008; Franz 2000; Franz 2002; Gannon 2001), many pump wearers report that adjusting their meal/snack bolus for a higher-than-usual consumption of protein and/or fat results in closer-to-target postprandial glucose levels (Ahern 1993; Chase 2002; Jones 2005; King 2007; Walsh 2012).

An insulin pump may provide three bolus delivery options: immediate, extended, and a combination of immediate and extended.

Extending a meal bolus over a period of time, ranging from 10 minutes to several hours, depending on the content of the food/meal or duration of eating time, is an option to achieve a target postprandial blood glucose level. A study in patients with type 1 diabetes comparing a dinner with equal amounts of carbohydrate and protein but different fat content (60 grams versus 10 grams) revealed that insulin requirements increased with the consumption of the higher-fat meal. These results indicate there is a need for alternative insulin dosing algorithms that are not based solely on carbohydrate content (Wolpert 2012). Extending a premeal bolus is an option for bolus delivery insulin. Pump manufacturers call this an extended or "square wave" bolus. The practice of extending a bolus delivery is a trial-and-error process and may take several weeks or months to master. The process requires experiments of bolus time durations and amounts and fastidious record keeping on the part of the user. CGM records provide assistance in developing time durations (Jones 2005). Another option is to divide or "split" the bolus, i.e., deliver a portion of it prior to the meal and the remaining portion "spread out" (extended) over several hours (combination or "dual wave" bolus). Both options enable the pumper to achieve desired postprandial glucose levels, but are dependent on the accuracy of the user's carb counting and individualized bolus calculator settings, including ICR(s), CF(s), blood glucose targets, and IOB.

Pump manufacturers provide a variety of extended bolus delivery choices. As of this writing, options range from 0–100% of the bolus delivered immediately with the remainder delivered in single-digit percentages anytime, varying from 10 minutes to 12 hours in 5- to 30-minute increments.

Pumps vary in their features and options, and manufacturers routinely develop and offer new options and improvements, so it is important for the HCP to be aware of the various models and features available.

*Examples of bolus doses (extended and combination):*
    2-ounce chocolate candy bar: 20 g carb, 1 g protein, 9 g fat
    Insulin-to-carbohydrate ratio: 1 u: 10 g
    Snack bolus: 2 units
    Extended bolus option: 2 units over 60 minutes

In this example, the pump user determined that the high fat content of the snack affected his 2-, 3-, and 4-h postprandial blood glucose readings.

Thanksgiving meal: 85 g carb, 42 g protein, 43 g fat
Insulin-to-carbohydrate ratio: 1 unit: 12 g
Meal bolus: 7.0 units
Combination bolus option: 3.5 units immediate bolus, 3.5 units extended over 2 h, 45 minutes

Pizza bolus: Combination bolus option: 35% immediately, 65% over 5 hours, 15 minutes.
Bolus dose amount varies, based on the grams of carbohydrate from the size and number of pizza slices consumed.

Pizza is a common food item/meal that often challenges the pump user, but with detailed records and trial-and-error experience using an extended or combination bolus feature, the pump user can experience postprandial glucose levels within their desired target range. In several studies, pizza with a fat content >36% was used to evaluate the use of a combination (dual wave) bolus with insulin lispro. Results from one study indicated that postprandial glucose excursions were lowest at 90–120 minutes when 70% of the bolus was delivered immediately and 30% was delivered extended over 2 hours (Chase 2002). Findings in another study showed that an equal split of 50% of the bolus delivered immediately and the remaining 50% delivered over 8 hours resulted in optimal glucose control with the lowest mean glucose level (Jones 2005).

Unfortunately, there are no published lists, charts, guidelines, pamphlets, articles, or books that can provide personalized or individualized bolus option amounts and time durations that are appropriate for each person. Every pump user is different and people react differently to foods consumed. To best determine appropriate customized boluses, the user should keep the following records for review and analysis. These factors will assist in making changes for bolus percentages and time durations:

- Preprandial glucose level
- Time of most recent bolus from previous meal/snack or correction
- Amount of most recent bolus from previous meal/snack or correction
- Duration of insulin action time remaining from previous meal/snack or correction (IOB/active insulin)
- Amount of carbohydrate to be consumed
- Amount of protein to be consumed

- Amount of fat to be consumed
- Amount of alcohol to be consumed
- Calculation of total bolus
- Type of bolus delivery: immediate, extended, or combination
- If extended bolus delivery, duration of time
- If combination bolus delivery, percentage of bolus delivered immediately and percentage of bolus delivered over time
- If combination bolus delivery, duration of time for extended portion of delivery
- One-, two-, three-, four-, and if appropriate, five- and six-hour postprandial glucose results.

Tips to help determine extended and combination bolus deliveries:

Trial and error will ultimately provide the appropriate amount of time duration for an extended bolus delivery. A good place to start when deciding on how long to extend a bolus is a 1-hour time duration. Based on postprandial results, the pump user can adjust the time duration by 10- or 15-minute increments until the desired target levels are achieved.

To determine how much of a combination bolus should be delivered immediately versus how much of the remainder should be delivered over time, many pump users start with a 50–50 split: 50% immediate, 50% over 1 hour. It can be a tedious process to determine exactly what should be adjusted: the split of the bolus amount, or the duration of time. Advise the pump user to change one factor at a time; otherwise, the person will not know what has affected the blood glucose results or what should be adjusted next. Some pump users prefer to first adjust the percentage of the split unit dose, especially if the postprandial glucose results are far from the desired target level. In other cases, pump users may choose to change the duration by 10- or 15-minute, 30-minute, or hourly time increments. Again, trial-and-error experiments and detailed record keeping are necessary (refer to "Sample Patient Insulin Pump Therapy Record" in Chapter 8).

Many other factors that affect blood glucose levels must also be taken into consideration, including IOB, physical activity, alcohol consumption, stress, hormones, etc. The process of determining an appropriate bolus option can take several weeks or months. However, once the pump user and HCP determine bolus options that work well, the individualized bolus options can be programmed into the pump, and target glucose levels can be more easily achieved and maintained.

## Bolus Considerations

A "missed" (omitted or forgotten) bolus also can be deleterious to a person's glucose level (Burdick 2004). Some pumps offer the convenience of setting reminders/alarms to remind the user to take certain actions. One alarm option on some pumps is the missed meal bolus alert alarm. This alarm can remind a person to deliver a bolus if they haven't taken a bolus within a specific time segment (such as between 6 a.m. and 10 a.m.). Many pump users find this to be extremely helpful, while others may tend to ignore the alarms (Chase 2002).

While it is important to teach insulin pump users to accurately calculate their carbohydrate consumption and bolus accordingly, there will be instances when "unexplained" glucose excursions or decreases occur. After basal rates have been checked, adjusted, and verified, and the clinician and/or pump user has factored in or accounted for the effects of hormone changes, stress, exercise, illness, and alcohol consumption, the insulin-to-carbohydrate ratio(s) may need to be adjusted. This is especially true when there are recurrent out-of-target glucose levels. Refer to "Insulin-to-Carbohydrate Ratio Adjustment" in Chapter 6 for information on how to adjust ICRs.

---

**Medications That May Warrant the Use of an Extended or Combination Bolus**

Some tricyclic antidepressants

Some anti-emetics

Opioids

Anticholinergics

---

# Alcohol

As a reminder, people with diabetes can choose to drink alcohol. From a health standpoint, the same guidelines that apply to the general population apply to people with diabetes. *The Dietary Guidelines for Americans* recommends limiting alcohol intake to two drinks per day for adult men and one drink a day for adult women. A drink is defined as 12 ounces of beer (5% alcohol), 5 ounces of wine (12% alcohol), or 1.5 ounces of 80 proof (40% alcohol) distilled spirits (U.S. Department of Agriculture and U.S. Department of Health and Human Services 2010). Each contains about 15 grams of alcohol (ADA 2008).

After consumption and even allowing for differences in size, women experience higher blood ethanol concentrations than men. This results in an increased bioavailability of alcohol resulting from decreased gastric first-pass metabolism and decreased gastric alcohol dehydrogenase activity. These factors may contribute to an enhanced susceptibility of females to the effects of alcohol (Frezza 1990).

Alcohol does not require insulin for metabolism. Pure alcohol, such as gin, rum, vodka, or whiskey contains calories but not carbohydrate. Moderate amounts of alcohol, when ingested with food, have minimal impact on plasma glucose (Koivisto 1993). However, alcohol can both increase and decrease blood glucose levels. An increase in blood glucose will occur if an excess of alcohol is consumed (Nanchahal 2000; Ben 1991; Feingold 1983). Additionally, any carbohydrate consumed with the alcohol, either in the alcoholic drink in the form of a "mixer," such as juice, tonic water, and other alcohol, or as a food, can increase blood glucose. Moderate (Lange 1991) or severe hypoglycemia (Arky 1968) has been reported in patients with diabetes after alcohol ingestion. Ingestion of moderate amounts of alcohol has also been shown to blunt the awareness of hypoglycemia in patients with type 1 diabetes (Kerr 1990).

As with any patient with diabetes, encourage the pump patient to ingest a form of carbohydrate when he/she consumes alcohol. When consuming an alcoholic beverage with a source of carbohydrate, such as a mixer, it may not be necessary to cover the carbohydrate in the mixer because of the potential hypoglycemic effect of the alcohol—trial and error may be necessary. Educate people that if they consume alcohol during the evening, the most common time for alcohol intake, they are at increased risk for hypoglycemia during the night or as late as the next morning (Richardson 2005). Alcohol can have a delayed blood glucose lowering effect, i.e., prevention of recovery, as much as 12 hours later due to its inhibition of gluconeogenesis (ADA 2008) and interference with the counterregulatory response to insulin-induced hypoglycemia (Turner 2001). For a pump patient, the use of a temporary decreased basal rate (example: 70–80% for several, up to 12, hours) after alcohol intake may be helpful.

Setting a reminder or alert to check blood glucose or consume carbohydrate while ingesting alcohol during a party, "happy hour," or a special occasion may also be helpful in preventing sudden or delayed hypoglycemia or hyperglycemia. The use of medical identification jewelry, informing family/friends of the potential for hypoglycemia, and additional SMBG while drinking are essential.

# Exercise and Physical Activity
GARY SCHEINER, MS, CDE

Physical activity has significant effects on people with diabetes. Increased blood flow to exercising muscle is accompanied by an increase in insulin-stimulated as well as non insulin-mediated glucose uptake (Thorell 1999). Concurrently, production of counterregulatory hormones (catecholamines, glucagon, cortisol, growth hormone) may increase abruptly during certain forms of exercise. As a result, glucose levels may rise, fall, or remain unchanged under different exercise conditions.

Although most studies have shown little impact on A1C levels for those with type 1 diabetes, the benefits of physical activity are far wider: weight control, functional capacity, reduced cardiovascular risk, and psychological well-being. For some insulin pump users, participation in physical activity is somewhat sporadic and related to leisure, chores, or work/school demands. For others, daily exercise is a part of an overall training/conditioning program. With persistence, expert guidance, and the benefit of peer support via social media, a growing number of insulin pump users are reaching for the highest levels of performance in a variety of both individual as well as group sports activities.

Diabetes, and certainly insulin pump use, should not limit one's ability to engage in virtually any form of physical activity. In fact, insulin pump use offers a number of unique advantages over injection therapy for the athlete with diabetes.

## Preventing Hypoglycemia

Most forms of low-to-moderate-intensity physical activity will increase insulin sensitivity and accelerate muscle cells' uptake of glucose. In a metabolically well-managed patient, this can produce an undesired drop in the blood glucose level. Some pump users believe that suspending or disconnecting from the pump will prevent hypoglycemia. However, given the time–action profile of rapid-acting insulin analogs used in pumps, eliminating basal insulin during the activity will have minimal effect on the glucose level during the activity. The most effective ways to prevent exercise-induced hypoglycemia are to reduce bolus insulin, increase food intake, or a combination of both (Rabasa-Lhoret 2001).

When physical activity is going to occur within 90 minutes after a meal, the best approach for preventing hypoglycemia is to reduce the mealtime bolus (DirectNet 2006; Sonnenberg 1990). Since both aspects of the bolus (the part given for food and the part given to correct an elevated glucose) are made more potent by physical activity, both need to be reduced. To accomplish this, reduce the usual mealtime bolus (based on the premeal glucose level and anticipated carbohydrate intake) by a percentage. The more intense and prolonged the activity, the greater the bolus reduction.

| Bolus Reduction ↘ | Short Duration (20–40 minutes) | Moderate Duration (40–60 minutes) | Long Duration (>60 minutes) |
|---|---|---|---|
| Low intensity | −10% | −20% | −30% |
| Moderate intensity | −25% | −33% | −50% |
| High intensity | −33% | −50% | −67% |

For example, if Florence plans a moderate-intensity 45-minute workout after breakfast, a 33% bolus reduction is likely in order. Her usual 6.0-unit dose would be reduced to 4.0 units.

When exercise is going to be performed before or between meals, reducing the bolus at the previous meal would only serve to drive the pre-workout glucose level very high. A better approach would be to take the normal bolus at the previous meal, and then snack prior to exercising—preferably by consuming high–glycemic index forms of carbohydrate such as cereal, crackers, or a sports drink (Coyle 1994).

The amount of the snack depends on the duration and intensity of the workout as well as the size of the individual. There is no way of knowing *exactly* how much will be needed, but the chart below should serve as a safe starting point.

| Weight of person with diabetes | Carbohydrate Replacement (g) Per 30 Minutes of Physical Activity | | | | |
| --- | --- | --- | --- | --- | --- |
| | 50 lb (23 kg) | 100 lb (45 kg) | 150 lb (68 kg) | 200 lb (91 kg) | 250 lb (114 kg) |
| Light Activity | 3 g | 5 g | 8 g | 10 g | 12 g |
| Moderate Activity | 5 g | 8 g | 10 g | 12 g | 15 g |
| Intense Activity | 8 g | 12 g | 18 g | 24 g | 30 g |

For example, if Bill weighs about 150 lb and is doing 90 minutes of intense yard work, he should consume about 18 g of carbohydrate before starting and every half hour during his yard work. Of course, if his pre-activity glucose level is above or below target, the amount of the initial snack should be adjusted accordingly.

## Basal Adjustment for Prolonged Activities

When engaging in relatively short periods of exercise (90 minutes or less), basal insulin adjustments tend to have little bearing on glucose levels. In fact, even short-term cessation of basal insulin delivery during exercise can produce post-exercise hyperglycemia (DirectNet 2006). It typically takes several hours for changes in basal insulin to have a noticeable effect. For prolonged activities (lasting 2 hours or more), basal insulin adjustments can be helpful for reducing the amount/frequency of snacks and preventing hypoglycemia. In most cases, a good starting point is to reduce the rate of basal insulin delivery by 50% using the temporary basal rate feature. With more intense activities, a reduction of 70–80% may be necessary to prevent a rapid decline in blood glucose.

To make the most of a temporary basal adjustment, it is best to start the adjustment 1 to 2 hours prior to the onset of prolonged physical activity (Frohnauer 2000). That way, when the activity begins, the level of basal insulin in the bloodstream will already be on the decline. It is best to end the temporary basal reduction shortly before the end of the activity so that the post-exercise insulin level returns to normal in a timely manner.

For example, if Barbara plans to ride her bike a long distance at a moderate pace, she can set a 50% temporary basal reduction 90 minutes before leaving. She should also snack periodically during her ride, but the amount and frequency of the snack should be much less than if she had not reduced her basal rate. A few miles before returning home, Barbara should end her temporary basal rate and return to her normal basal rate setting.

## Delayed Effects

Exhaustive forms of exercise, such as prolonged/intense aerobic activities and maximal strength training, deplete muscle glycogen stores and greatly increase muscle sensitivity to insulin. This combination can cause blood glucose to drop several hours after cessation of the activity—a phenomenon called "delayed-onset hypoglycemia" (MacDonald 1987; Price 1994).

Anyone who uses insulin can prevent a delayed fall in blood glucose by consuming slow-digesting (low–glycemic index) carbohydrate without compensatory insulin. However, by having the ability to temporarily reduce basal insulin levels, insulin pump users are in a unique position to prevent delayed-onset hypoglycemia. Once a pattern of delayed glucose lowering is detected, patients can usually prevent further bouts of hypoglycemia through a modest 20–30% temporary basal insulin reduction. The adjustment should be made following the activity, and set for a duration that lasts until the glucose drop normally occurs.

For example, Tom finds that his glucose level drops overnight after he plays full-court basketball during the day. To prevent this delayed drop, he can set a 25% basal decrease that runs from after basketball until the middle of the night.

## Managing Exercise-induced Hyperglycemia

Glucose regulation involves a complex interaction between the factors that raise blood glucose (carbohydrate in the diet and counterregulatory hormones) and the factors that lower it (insulin and physical activity). Some forms of exercise induce a dramatic increase in stress hormones, resulting in an acute rise in blood glucose (Mitchell 1988). Examples include:

- Weight lifting, particularly when working muscles to the point of fatigue
- Sports that involve intermittent "bursts" of activity such as softball, golf, or martial arts
- Maximal sprints in events such as running, swimming, and rowing
- Events where performance is being judged, such as gymnastics or figure skating
- Sports in which winning is the primary objective

For those who detect a consistent rise in their blood glucose during certain activities, the solution is to take extra insulin in preparation for the event. Because physical activity makes the body more sensitive to insulin, a reasonable pre-activity bolus is equal to 50% of the amount required to offset the expected rise, administered 30–60 minutes before exercising.

For example, if Doris's glucose tends to rise 100 mg/dl when she runs a 5 k race and her sensitivity to insulin (correction factor) is 50 mg/dl, she would normally require a 2-unit bolus to offset the adrenaline-induced blood glucose rise. Instead, she takes 1 unit an hour prior to the run and monitors her glucose level closely.

Another potential source of rising glucose during exercise is a lack of working insulin in the body. Because insulin pump users do not take long-acting insulin, any problem with insulin delivery, absorption, or potency can result in significant insulin deficiency in just a few hours. Without sufficient insulin to meet the body's basic metabolic needs, exercise will usually cause a rapid glucose rise and, potentially, progression toward diabetic ketoacidosis (DKA).

For this reason, pump users should check their blood (or urine, if a blood ketone meter is unavailable) for ketones whenever glucose levels are inexplicably elevated prior to exercise. Patients should be instructed to treat the hyperglycemia and ketones according to standard procedure (typically administering insulin via injection, hydrating, and changing the pump's infusion set) and postponing exercise until ketones have cleared and the glucose level returns to an acceptable range (American Diabetes Association 2013, 2004).

In the absence of ketones, it is not usually dangerous to exercise with a high glucose level. Performance may not be optimal, but the risk to the patient is minimal. The best option is to administer a bolus equal to half of the usual correction dose and hydrate adequately.

Extended disconnection (>90 minutes) from a pump can also cause a rise in the glucose level during or immediately following exercise. Many pump users choose to temporarily disconnect from the pump during sports that involve rough contact, jarring movements, or exposure to water. Doing so for less than 90 minutes rarely presents a problem; it is not usually necessary to "replace" any of the missed basal insulin. However, for longer periods of disconnection, the patient should be instructed to reconnect hourly and administer a bolus equal to 50% of the usual basal rate.

For example, Sara prefers to disconnect from her pump while swimming and playing at the beach. Given that her usual basal rate is 0.6 units/hr, she reconnects hourly, delivers a bolus of 0.3 units, and then promptly disconnects.

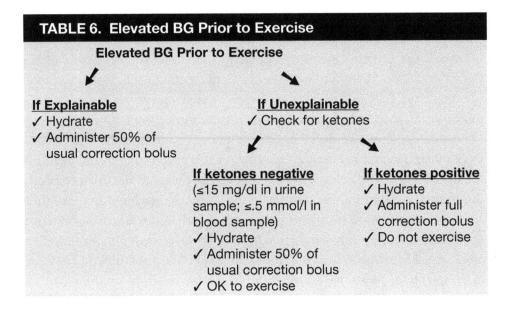

**TABLE 6. Elevated BG Prior to Exercise**

Elevated BG Prior to Exercise

**If Explainable**
✓ Hydrate
✓ Administer 50% of
   usual correction bolus

**If Unexplainable**
✓ Check for ketones

**If ketones negative**
(≤15 mg/dl in urine
sample; ≤.5 mmol/l in
blood sample)
✓ Hydrate
✓ Administer 50% of
   usual correction bolus
✓ OK to exercise

**If ketones positive**
✓ Hydrate
✓ Administer full
   correction bolus
✓ Do not exercise

When prolonged or intense activities preclude hourly reconnection to the pump, an *untethered program* may be utilized. This involves injecting a small dose of long-acting basal insulin in the morning and utilizing a secondary/reduced basal program on the pump for the next 24 hours. This approach allows for safe disconnection for extended periods of time, particularly during the daytime hours when the basal rate is usually at its lowest.

## Infusion Set Practices

For every insulin pump user, the infusion set should be matched to the individual's needs. Patients who participate in high-impact sports activities should be advised to use a flexible Teflon cannula rather than a metal/steel needle to prevent potential discomfort and injury at the infusion site. Angled infusion sets work best for most lean athletes, as the angled orientation reduces the chances of penetrating or poking the underlying muscle wall. The clear window on the angled sets allow rapid detection of site irritation and bleeding, and the longer cannula on an angled set is less likely to accidentally pull out of the skin compared to a shorter cannula that is inserted in a perpendicular fashion.

Some patients have difficulty keeping their pump infusion set in place when exercising. Perspiration and rapid movements can cause the set to come loose or cause irritation below the skin. One of the best strategies for avoiding these types of problems is to wear the set on the buttocks, where there is ample subcutaneous fat, the skin does not move/stretch excessively, perspiration is minimal, and there is typically a tight garment covering the site.

Some athletes also find it helpful to place an adhesive dressing such as IV-3000 or Tegaderm over the infusion set. Cutting a hole in the center of the dressing before placing it over the set allows access to the usual connect/disconnect mechanism (for those who use a set that disconnects at the infusion site). If adhesion problems persist, a topical adhesive such as Mastisol applied around the point of insertion prior to set placement provides excellent adherence (Medtronic 2011). Refer to "Infusion Site and Tubing Concerns" in Chapter 6 for additional information. One other potential solution, particularly for those who perspire excessively, is use of a strong antiperspirant such as Hypercare—a prescription-only antiperspirant containing a high concentration of aluminum chloride (20%). Applying Hypercare the night before inserting an infusion set works well for most patients. Many also report significantly less site itching, redness, and irritation when the skin does not perspire.

## Wearing the Pump During Exercise

Insulin pumps are made to withstand a considerable amount of impact. The majority of experienced pump users have found that insulin pumps do not interfere with most forms of sports activities. To that end, a number of excellent options exist for wearing the pump during exercise. If the standard clip will not hold the pump in place well enough, or if extra stability or protection is sought, a variety of pump accessories are available. These include the *SportPak* (Unique Pump Accessories) and *Zipps* (Pump Wear Inc.). Spandex belts with pump-sized pockets that fit securely around the arm, thigh, or calf are also available.

Waterproof or water-resistant pumps can be used in depths ranging from 8 to 12 feet for varying periods of time. Always check the manufacturer's pump specs and recommendations for use in and around water. For waterproofing pumps that are not already watertight, pumpers can utilize a case such as the AquaPac (AquaPac International Ltd). This clear, flexible case allows the pump to be programmed while inside, and features a pass-through port for the pump tubing. Of course, this is not necessary with waterproof pumps and "patch"-type pumps.

Occasionally, exercise may take place under extreme conditions. High ambient temperature during exercise may lead to set adhesion problems; it can also contribute to insulin breakdown (Eli Lilly 2011, Novo Nordisk 2002–2011, sanofi-aventis 2009). Cold temperatures are not usually an issue as long as the pump is worn close to the body, but heat can lead to denaturing of insulin and hyperglycemia. When exercising at temperatures above 86°F, advise patients to shield their pump and tubing from direct sunlight. With prolonged exposure to warm temperatures, it may be necessary to change the pump cartridge/reservoir and tubing more frequently than usual. If exposure to high temperatures (>98°F) is unavoidable, use of an insulated cooling pouch such as the Frio Pump Wallet (Frio Ltd) is an effective way to avoid insulin spoilage.

**Parameters for the Patient to Consider When Exercising**

- The type, intensity, and duration of the exercise
- Time of day
- Glucose level at start of exercise
- Prior experiences with similar types of exercise
- Basal rate during the exercise session
- Amount of bolus insulin on board
- Time of last meal/snack
- Infusion set placement location
- Hydration level

# Intimacy/Sexual Activity

Remind the patient that increased physical activity, including intimacy, may necessitate a decreased amount of insulin. Depending on the duration of intimacy, a decreased basal rate may be necessary for a few hours; trial and error will determine this information. CGM may also be useful to determine if there is a need to change the basal rate(s) during and/or after sexual activity. To wear the pump or not during intimacy is the patient's choice. Wearing a pod-type or "tubeless" pump may present less of a challenge than a pump with tubing. If the patient wants to keep their non-pod-style pump connected, a longer infusion set tubing can be considered. The pump wearer can place the pump freely in the bed, under or next to a pillow, or attached to clothing using a clip or placed in a pocket.

If the pump user chooses to temporarily disconnect his or her pump or infusion set for several hours, advise the patient to deliver a compensatory bolus before removing the pump. For example, if the basal rate is 0.6 units/h and the pump will be removed for 1.5 h, the compensatory bolus would be 0.9 units delivered before disconnecting or removing the pump. The patient should be reminded to reconnect his or her infusion set and pump (or tubeless pump), especially before falling asleep. If the patient prefers to disconnect their pump, use of the "suspend" function on the pump and the accompanying alarm will alert the patient to reconnect the pump, but some people may find the alarm annoying or bothersome. When reconnecting a pump with tubing, the infusion site should always be checked to make certain the set base has remained intact.

# Managing Sick Days and Medical Procedures
WITH NICHOLAS B. ARGENTO, MD

The pump patient uses the same basic sick day guidelines that apply to anyone using insulin:

- Check and record the results of blood glucose more frequently.
- If blood glucose exceeds 240 mg/dl on two occasions, check ketones.
- Do not decrease basal insulin doses unless hypoglycemia develops; basal rates may need to be increased 20–50% for the duration of the illness. Mild colds, the flu, and dental surgery may require smaller temporary increases (10–20%) or other adjustments in basal rates.
- Increase noncaloric fluids.
- If lack of appetite or vomiting exists, substitute caloric-/carbohydrate-containing fluids for solid foods, if tolerated.
- Call physician or appropriate healthcare professional if hyperglycemia, nausea, vomiting, or diarrhea persists for >4 h; if there is a fever >100°F; if there are moderate to large ketones present in the urine; or if hypoglycemia is developing.

Patients should know how to program their pump for temporary rate changes. Remind the patient that if basal rates are set correctly, the omission of food should not result in hypoglycemia. On the contrary, hyperglycemia may occur rapidly during illness and, if untreated, lead to ketosis and ketoacidosis. Go over the patient's plan of action for severe illness or emergency. Emphasize to the patient the need to continue to check their blood glucose frequently, even if they are not eating. Provide guidelines to the patient for temporary basal rate increases, including duration and percentages of change. *Keep in mind that pump manufacturer customer support staff or per diem CDEs cannot provide medical treatment guidelines to insulin pump therapy patients.*

During hospitalization, continuation of pump therapy is at the discretion of the admitting physician and may require limited staff training. All patients on pumps admitted to a hospital should have an endocrine consult. Some hospitals have protocols for the admission of insulin pump therapy patients. Psychiatric admissions may necessitate removal of the pump and a return to injection therapy that can be monitored and administered by the hospital staff. But in general, a pump patient admitted for a nonpsychiatric reason might do better by staying on pump therapy as long as the patient: is alert and is not sedated; knows how to change their pump settings; is physically able to operate the pump, perform infusion set changes, and all necessary pump supplies are available and the pump is in good working order; does not need high doses of corticosteroids; and does not need hyperalimentation. If the blood glucose cannot be adequately controlled on pump therapy, then the pump should be discontinued and alternative insulin replacement started. Patients who are to be switched from using their insulin pump and are not started on IV insulin should be changed to a basal-bolus regimen that takes into consideration using the patient's basal rates, insulin-to-carbohydrate ratio(s) and correction factor(s) as appropriate. Refer to Chapter 8, Forms and Resources, Patient Guidelines, Checklists, and Forms, for a suggested letter for the patient to present to the admitting physician on the day of admission.

Close communication between the attending physician and patient is essential if pump therapy is to be continued in a hospital setting. Recent blood glucose results will need to be reviewed. The physician will need to advise what treatments the patient is getting and how they are likely to affect insulin needs, and what the plans are in terms of nutritional intake. Only then can decisions be made on any changes in pump settings. It is critical that the patient and attending staff understand that if the pump is removed, the attending physician must properly replace the basal rate plus any required nutritional and correction factor insulin, and not just put the patient on a "sliding scale," which can result in the development of severe hyperglycemia or even iatrogenic diabetic ketoacidosis.

Advise the patient to discuss a hospital admission with the admitting physician. Remind the patient that the hospital will not have or be able to provide any pump supplies and to bring a supply of infusion sets, cartridges/reservoirs, batteries, infusion set prep products, clips or cases, etc., as appropriate. If the hospital does not have in a vial the type of insulin that the patient uses in their pump, the patient may need to supply the insulin as well. If the patient uses prefilled pump cartridges, those would need to be supplied by the patient. The patient should be prepared to provide their basal rates, insulin-to-carb ratio(s), correction factor(s), and total daily dose. Additionally, although the hospital will perform blood glucose checks with their own system, the patient who checks more frequently than before meals and at bedtime may want to bring their own glucose meter and supplies. Medical identification (bracelet, necklace) is advised.

For outpatient procedures and surgeries, including dental surgery, pump therapy is usually continued, and the patient and/or the healthcare team must provide basic information to the procedure or surgical staff team. Advise your patient that hospital staff and most physicians know little or nothing about an insulin pump. This information may include the need to tape or secure the pump to the hospital gown, what to do or who to call if the pump alarm sounds during the procedure, and an alternative insulin delivery plan if the pump must be removed. For any surgery, remind the patient to check the pump's settings and temporarily disable alerts and alarms for missed meal bolus, set/site change reminder, check blood glucose, automatic basal suspend, etc., for the time periods before, during, and while in the recovery room. If the patient uses an automatic basal suspend function, care should be taken to be sure that the pump is not shut off unintentionally in the peri-operative period.

Insulin pumps can be damaged by exposure to strong magnetic fields or X-rays. Consequently, an insulin pump, including the pod used with a tubeless pump, should be removed when a patient needs X-rays, CT scans, or MRI scans. For questions about the safety of exposure to other types of radiation, encourage the pump user to check with their pump manufacturer (by viewing the information on the manufacturer's website or calling the customer service patient support line) for specific recommendations.

# Stress
Nicholas B. Argento, MD

Stress, though a normal part of life, can cause erratic glucose responses. Stressors can be positive and negative, short- or long-term, and can affect a person's ability to achieve and maintain good control. Inadequate sleep, too much food, inactivity, and the release of counterregulatory hormones can all increase the blood glucose level. Stress from illness or infection raises blood glucose levels (refer to preceding information regarding illness). Many patients with diabetes report significant psychological stress related to increased self-care demands, increased financial costs, fear of both short- and long-term complications, and dealing with established complications. Psychological stress can raise blood glucose levels, directly through higher counterregulatory hormone levels, or indirectly through decreased adherence to diabetes-related self-care recommendations. Frequent or chronic stress can be associated with poorer blood glucose control in patients with diabetes, which may improve with therapy (Ismail 2004). People cope with stress in different ways, including seeking support from family, friends, a religious community, or support group, as well as exercise, relaxation techniques, and psychological counseling. Keep in mind that some people may use alcohol or illicit drugs, and these coping mechanisms will add to erratic blood glucose control.

While using the correction factor on a smart pump can help with acute stress, stress that is more chronic may call for using higher basal rates during those periods. For example, it might be appropriate for a patient to use a higher basal rate during the work week if s/he felt their job was stressful and review of blood glucose data indicated consistently higher blood glucoses, or the need for higher insulin dosing, during those times. Most pumps allow multiple basal profiles to be programmed, which can help, though the patient needs to remember to change the active basal profile to the appropriate basal profile when the situation has changed. An alternative approach might be to use a time-limited temporary basal rate when the patient is in a situation s/he knows is likely to increase their blood glucose level. Recommending that boluses (combined carbohydrate and correction insulin) be manually increased, such as increasing the recommended bolus by one-third during such times, can be an effective strategy, but would require the patient to override smart pump recommendations. Such a recommendation has the advantage of requiring the patient to actively consider whether to increase the bolus at that time. In contrast, if the patient changes his/her bolus settings and forgets to switch them back when the stress has resolved, then the recommended boluses will be too large, which could lead to hypoglycemia.

# Travel
WITH NICHOLAS B. ARGENTO, MD

Traveling takes even more foresight and planning on the part of the pump patient. The upside is that an insulin pump makes travel easier and more enjoyable because of the enhanced ability to adapt to time changes and altered meal schedules. When travel includes sedentary activity that is longer than usual, the patient may need a temporary increase in basal rates. A 10–20% (110–120% of the basal rate) increase may be appropriate (Kaufman 2012).

In addition to packing daily supplies, plus 50% more for emergencies or delayed return, advise the patient to have:

- Spare pump, if available. Some pump companies provide a loaner pump for travel to foreign or remote areas, or for cruises. The pump manufacturer can also provide information on the availability of their pump or pump supplies in foreign countries similar or identical to their product(s) in the U.S. but marketed under a different name internationally.
- Spare glucose meter and supplies, if available
- Readily available treatment for hypoglycemia. Examples include: glucose tablets, soft non-chocolate candy, hard sugary candies, and fruit juice in small boxes. Items purchased post–security screening in U.S. airports can be carried on a plane, but advise patients to check with the Transportation Security Administration (TSA) regarding current regulations for liquids necessary for medical treatment.
- Puncture-proof container for used lancets and infusion sets. Empty shampoo bottles work well.
- Ketone check strips

- Glucagon treatment, which travel partner(s) should know how to use
- Extra vial(s) of rapid-acting insulin in the original box with label and syringes
- Basal (intermediate- or long-acting) insulin pen/pen needles or vial/ syringes in the original box with prescription label
- Copy of an appropriate basal-bolus injection therapy regimen
- Prescriptions for insulin and other medications, including a list of current medications with dosages and frequency (Note: Prescriptions for liquid medications, such as insulin, may not be acceptable by security personnel due to forgery concerns, but may be useful in case of an emergency. Prescriptions for pump supplies also may not be helpful, since pump supplies are usually not available locally.)
- Extra prescription eyeglasses
- For remote areas, the name, address, and phone number of the nearest medical facility

All (travel) pump and medical items should be packed in carry-on luggage, and, if possible, divided between travel partners. Automobile, train, and airline travel may require refrigeration of insulin, depending on the length of the trip and storage conditions. Since insulin in a vial is stable at room temperature for 28 days, most patients can be reassured that they will not need access to refrigeration as long as the insulin will not be exposed to extreme temperatures.

An insulin pump will draw some scrutiny when going through security checkpoints. Most rail and airline security personnel are familiar with an insulin pump but may require the patient to show the pump.

Patients who are traveling by air should be instructed to inform security personnel that they are wearing an insulin pump/CGM device, that it cannot be easily removed, and be aware that they might possibly be subjected to secondary search procedures. Please review the information from the Transportation Security Administration below.

The low-dose X-rays involved in screening (X-rays or total body scanners) may or may not harm an insulin pump, or other diabetes devices like continuous glucose monitors and meters.

Pump manufactures make different recommendations. Some pump manufacturer's user guides state that security systems used in airports should not affect pump function. However, when various pump company websites were accessed on 10 February 2013, several companies recommended that their pumps not be subjected to X-ray or whole body scanners, but noted that magnetic walk-through with secondary inspection was safe. One company's website recommended that their compatible CGM device also has the same restrictions, though it can be used while in flight. Several pump manufacturers noted that the glucose meter link feature should be turned off while in flight. A CGM manufacturer had no restriction on airport screening in the user guide of one of their models, but in a newer model's user guide, the company makes the recommendation that the system not be put through X-ray systems. The manufacturer notes that magnetic detectors and handwanding are safe and they recommend requesting visual inspection of the CGM system. That manufacturer also noted that it is okay to use the system while in flight. It is important to emphasize to patients that prior to airline or rail travel, the patient should check with their pump/CGM device manufacturer for the latest recommendations regarding X-ray screening of the pump/CGM device. They should also check the TSA website.

The following information was obtained from the Transportation Security Administration (TSA) regarding people with diabetes flying within the United States (TSA updated 28 January 2013). The TSA Cares Help Line (toll free, 1–855–787–2227) is available to assist travelers with disabilities and medical conditions. The TSA recommends that passengers call 72 hours prior to traveling with questions about screening policies, procedures and what to expect at the security checkpoint. Calling 72 hours in advance of travel will also provide the TSA the opportunity to coordinate checkpoint support with a TSA Customer Service Manager located at the airport when necessary. The hours of operation for the TSA Cares helpline are Monday through Friday 8 a.m.–11 p.m. EST and weekends and holidays 9 a.m.–8 p.m. EST.

Diabetes-related supplies, equipment, and medication, including liquids, are allowed through the security checkpoint after they have been properly screened by X-ray or hand inspection. Passengers should separate these items from other belongings and declare them to the security officer before screening begins.

Liquids, gels, and aerosols are screened by X-ray; medically necessary items in excess of 3.4 ounces will receive additional screening. A passenger could be asked to open the liquid or gel for additional screening. The TSA will not touch the liquid or gel during this process. If the passenger doesn't want a liquid, gel, or aerosol X-rayed or opened for additional screening, s/he should inform the officer before screening begins. Additional screening of the passenger and their property may be required and may include a patdown.

Accessories required to keep medically necessary liquids, gels, and aerosols cool, such as freezer packs or frozen gel pack, are permitted through the screening checkpoint and may be subject to additional screening. These accessories are treated as liquids unless they are frozen solid at the checkpoint. If these accessories are partially frozen or slushy, they are subject to the same screening as other liquids and gels.

A passenger who uses an insulin pump can be screened without disconnecting from the pump. The passenger should inform the officer conducting the screening about the pump before the screening process begins. Screening can be conducted using imaging technology, a metal detector, or a thorough patdown. A passenger can request to be screened by patdown in lieu of imaging technology.

Regardless of whether the passenger is screened using imaging technology or metal detector, the passenger's insulin pump is subject to additional screening. Under most circumstances, this will include the passenger conducting a self-patdown of the insulin pump followed by an explosive trace detection sampling (swabbing the device and hands).

Additionally, the American Diabetes Association's *Fact Sheet— Air Travel and Diabetes* (American Diabetes Association 2012) states: Examples of items that are permitted through security:

■ Insulin- and insulin-loaded dispensing products (vials or box of individual vials, jet injectors, biojectors, epipens, infusers, and preloaded syringes)

■ Unlimited number of unused syringes when accompanied by insulin or other injectable medication

■ Lancets, blood glucose meters, blood glucose meter test strips, alcohol swabs, meter-testing solutions

■ Insulin pump and insulin pump supplies (cleaning agents, batteries, plastic tubing, infusion kit, catheter, and needle)—insulin pumps and supplies must be accompanied by insulin

■ Glucagon emergency kit

■ Urine ketone test strips

■ Unlimited number of used syringes when transported in sharps disposal container or other similar hard-surface container

■ Sharps disposal containers/similar hard-surface disposal container for storing used syringes and test strips

■ Liquids (to include water, juice, or liquid nutrition) or gels

■ Continuous blood glucose monitors

■ All diabetes-related medication, equipment, and supplies

The question of how commercial airline cabin pressure changes may affect insulin pump delivery has received scrutiny. King and associates evaluated insulin pumps made by two different companies in a study that looked at both simulated and actual plane trips. They reported that insulin pumps may deliver an excess of 1.0–1.4 units insulin on ascent, and suck back 0.58 to 0.89 units on descent, in both cases as a result of the effect of the changes in cabin pressure on gas behavior. Further, they simulated catastrophic decompression, a fortunately rare event, but one reported to occur about 40 to

50 times a year, and found a large bolus of about 8 units was delivered. They recommended the following (King 2011a):

■ The pump cartridge/reservoir should contain a volume of 1.5 ml (150 units) or less, since the magnitude of the effect is larger with larger volumes.
■ The pump patient should disconnect the pump before ascent, then remove any air bubbles once at cruising altitude (e.g. prime while disconnected), which should be 30 minutes later, then reconnect the infusion set.
■ On descent, once on the ground, the patient should disconnect, prime two units, then reconnect the infusion set.
■ In the event of a catastrophic decompression, the patient should disconnect the pump.

Questions have been raised about both the necessity and practicality of these recommendations, and concerns expressed about the possibility of the patient not reconnecting, which could lead to hyperglycemia, or even ketoacidosis (Hirsch 2011). Not all pumps were studied, so no definite conclusions can be drawn. It is unclear how one would institute these recommendations with currently available patch pumps. If one were to implement these recommendations, emphasize to the patient that they must not forget to reconnect the pump. For short flights, it is probably not necessary to disconnect, since the overdose with ascent and underdose after descent are similar in magnitude. Since pumps alarm when they are in the suspend mode, the use of the suspend function while detached should serve to remind the patient that they are disconnected, as long as the patient can hear the alarm or feel the vibration alert, which may be an issue for some. While it does not seem very likely that a patient exposed to the trauma of a catastrophic decompression would remember to quickly disconnect their pump, it has been pointed out that even if they did not do so, it would be important for them to understand that they would have been bolused with a large dose of insulin, so that they could take corrective action (King 2011b).

When changing time zones, it is best to keep the pump on local time while traveling and reset the pump clock upon arrival at the new destination. A reasonable strategy is to change all devices (pump, meter, and CGM) at the same time to the new local time upon arrival. For time changes of 1 to 2 h, it may not be necessary to make basal rate adjustments. Anecdotally, some well-traveled experienced pumpers report that changing the pump clock gradually to "catch up" with the body's change in circadian rhythm works well. If the basal rates vary dramatically over 24 hours (e.g., much higher basal rate for the dawn phenomenon) and there are several time zone changes, an option is to make gradual changes in steps by 1 to 2 hours each day to better match the body's diurnal clock change (Wolpert 2002). A 6-hour time zone change, for example, could be adjusted over 3 days with 2-hour adjustments each day. Although successfully used by some well-experienced pumpers, exercise caution with this tactic, as it can be confusing to the patient and may complicate the travel experience. It is most important that the daytime and nighttime basal rates be consistent with the destination time. Bolus doses should be administered as usual, and frequent SMBG is essential. Changes in ICRs and correction factor(s) should not be necessary. However, the patient would need to consider whether they need to reduce a bolus if the travel involves more exertion than normal, or increase it if the travel involves less activity than normal.

# Weight Change
Nicholas B. Argento, MD

Weight gain is a well-known complication of intensive therapy in type 1 diabetes, as is an increase in the risk of hypoglycemia (Diabetes Control and Complications Trial Research Group 1993). An increased frequency of hypoglycemia will lead to more ingestion of the extra calories needed for hypoglycemia treatment. Some patients may feel more freedom to eat "forbidden" foods that they previously avoided due to the greater dietary flexibility that can accompany insulin pump therapy. Reducing the average blood glucose will lead to reduced glucosuria, which could lead to retaining a greater proportion of ingested calories, a factor that will lead to weight gain unless caloric intake is cut 250–300 calories per day (Delahanty 1993). Whether there are more fundamental reasons for the weight gain associated with intensified therapy, such as increased peripheral insulin levels causing increased energy uptake by peripheral adipose tissue, is not clear. It should also be stated that increasing weight and rising obesity rates are a problem not just for those with diabetes, but for the population as a whole. There are societal and dietary factors that are promoting weight gain in those without diabetes (Swinburn 2011), and patients with diabetes are not immune to these factors.

Strategies that might help minimize weight gain include:

- emphasizing reduced portion sizes
- emphasizing to the patient not to overtreat hypoglycemic episodes with excessive carbohydrate. Encourage use of the "Rule of 15" (15 g carbohydrate, recheck in 15 minutes, repeat as necessary)
- dietary education and planning to include total calorie targets appropriate to either maintain or lose weight
- increasing exercise, which might be easier to manage with less hypoglycemia by taking advantage of pump features like setting a lower temporary basal rate before or during exercise, or reducing insulin coverage of carbohydrates ingested before exercise
- use of pramlintide in selected patients (Ratner 2004)

Eating disorders are relatively common in patients with diabetes, especially in adolescents and young adults (Rodin 1991) and can be associated with higher A1C levels (Mannucci 1995). Fear of weight gain can lead to the patient purposely omitting or reducing doses of insulin. Binge eating without covering the carbohydrate with insulin has been referred to as "diabulemia." Such patients can be particularly challenging. Careful review of pump downloads can reveal evidence of minimal or absent bolusing, or prolonged periods of basal suspension, though one would not be able to detect binge eating without bolusing unless continuous glucose monitoring is in use. Probing for evidence of an eating disorder, and appropriate referral for psychological and dietary counseling, would be indicated in such patients.

Significant weight loss would be expected to reduce the need for basal insulin and reduce bolus ratios. Unintended weight loss in a patient with type 1 diabetes should prompt consideration of possible autoimmune causes of weight loss such as hyperthyroidism, adrenal insufficiency, and celiac disease, in addition to any other appropriate workup that would be indicated for a patient without diabetes who had unintended weight loss.

# Menses, Peri-menopause, and Menopause
Nicholas B. Argento, MD

Many menstruating women note changes in their blood glucose levels at different times during the menstrual cycle, particularly an increased need for insulin the week before and at the start of menses, times when one would expect higher reproductive hormone levels (Sherman 1975). A pump allows the use of different basal profiles, as noted above, and it might be helpful to use higher basal rates during the premenstrual period. However, the patient would need to remember to change the basal profile when she starts to see lower insulin needs. Failure to do so could lead to hypoglycemia, and for this reason this approach is not advisable in all patients. An alternative strategy would be for the patient to use the temporary basal rate function on successive days. This approach has the advantage of being time limited, and therefore its continuation requires an active decision. Manually increasing the recommended bolus by one-quarter to one-half the total, as with stress, is also helpful, and has the advantage of requiring an active decision each time a bolus is altered. Women with type 1 diabetes have been reported to have higher rates of delayed menarche, the earlier onset of menopause, and more menstrual irregularities (Strotmeyer 2003) than women without type 1 diabetes; the last of these factors would make cyclic blood glucose changes less predictable.

Use of oral contraceptives can increase insulin resistance (Kraus 1992), thus requiring an increase in insulin pump basal and bolus settings, at least while active drug is being administered. Use of the lower-estrogen-dose agents is preferable because they induce less insulin resistance (Kraus1992). There are conflicting reports of the effects of hormone replacement therapy (HRT) on glucose homeostasis in post-menopausal women, though the use of post-menopausal HRT has been reported not to alter the A1C in healthy women (Okada 2003). Increased glucose monitoring when starting HRT in woman with diabetes would seem to be prudent.

# Pregnancy
Nicholas B. Argento, MD

It is well recognized that tight glycemic control during a pregnancy complicated by diabetes can reduce the frequency of fetal malformations, obstetrical complications, and fetal morbidity, and that preventing fetal malformations requires tight control early in pregnancy (Kitzmiller 1996). Prior to pregnancy, the target A1C should be as close to normal as possible as allowed by hypogly-cemia, utilizing an intensive insulin regimen (Kitzmiller 2008), including use of an insulin pump. If a pump is to be used, it is preferable that the patient be started pre-pregnancy when possible, to allow safer adjustment to pump ther-apy. A pump can be started during pregnancy, but extremely close monitoring and intensive support during the start-up procedure would be needed.

Full discussion of the topic of pregestational diabetes is beyond the scope of this book. The reader is referred to the most recent American Diabetes Asso-ciation (ADA) Consensus Statement, which as of this printing was in May 2008 (Kitzmiller 2008), for full consideration of the topic. The ADA's consensus pan-el's current recommendations for insulin treatment for pregestational diabetes during pregnancy include using basal-bolus therapy with either:

- multiple injections of a rapid-acting insulin analog that has randomized control trials (RCTs) showing safety and effectiveness in pregnancy, which as of now include insulin aspart and insulin lispro, along with NPH insulin 2 to 3 times a day*, or
- use of an insulin pump, using insulin aspart or insulin lispro, with expert opinion being that these analogs could allow better control of postpran-dial hyperglycemia with less hypoglycemia, versus using regular insulin.

*Of note, since the publication of the ADA Consensus Statement in 2008, insulin detemir received an FDA pregnancy category B rating in April 2012 ([www.novonordisk-us.com] NovoNordisk 2012). As of this writing, insulin glulisine and insulin glargine are rated FDA pregnancy category C ([www.sanofi.us] sanofi aventis 2007; sanofi aventis 2009).

Insulin pump therapy has not been shown to have better outcomes ver-sus multiple daily injections for the mother or fetus in RCTs, but it was noted that "the multiple adjustable basal rates offered by continuous subcutaneous insulin action (CSII) can be especially useful for patients with daytime or noc-turnal hypoglycemia or a prominent dawn phenomenon (increased insulin requirement between 4:00 a.m. and 8:00 a.m.)." It was also noted that the potential for marked hyperglycemia and ketoacidosis due to insulin infusion interruption mandated that the patient be well trained in managing the insulin pump (Kitzmiller 2008), a point that cannot be overemphasized.

In the view of many clinicians, insulin pump therapy is ideal during pregnancy and should be considered in the preconception period when the goal is to intensify management, lower A1C, reduce hypoglycemia, and stabilize glucose levels to create the best outcomes for the mother and the baby (Kaufman 2012). Pump therapy may be especially useful during the first trimester when morning sickness is most prevalent. The patient's basal rate(s) can maintain normoglycemia and the patient can bolus her prandial insulin after consuming the food she was able to tolerate, rather than bolus before eating and risking hypoglycemia due to the inability to hold down her food.

The recommended targets for glucose control during pregnancy include fasting and premeal blood glucose levels of 60–99 mg/dl and 1-hour postprandial blood glucoses below 130 mg/dl, an average blood glucose of below 110 mg/dl, and an A1C below 6.0%, or higher values if those goals cannot be achieved with an acceptable risk of hypoglycemia. The need for insulin increases substantially in the first trimester, falls in the late first trimester, and then increases steadily until the end of the third trimester. SMBG monitoring daily before meals, 1 hour after meals, before bed, and occasionally at 2 to 3 a.m. is needed (Kitzmiller 2008).

Use of a pump facilitates patient compliance with the need for frequent dosing of insulin, including with snacks, and also allows more flexible adjustment of basal rates. Close follow-up and at least twice-weekly reassessment of blood glucose results are necessary to guide the increase in all pump rates that will be needed as pregnancy progresses. The need to get the postmeal blood glucose under 130 mg/dl often necessitates dosing a rapid-acting insulin analog 20 minutes before a meal, a finding that should not be surprising since nonpregnant patients have also been shown to achieve better postprandial blood glucose control by dosing a rapid-acting insulin analog 20 minutes ahead of the meal (Corey 2010). It is important to emphasize to the patient that she should not bolus ahead if she is hypoglycemic pre-meal, and that it is important that she not allow a 20-minute delay to become more prolonged, which would increase the risk of hypoglycemia. The need for strict carbohydrate counting, avoiding high-glycemic foods like boxed cereals and fruit juice, and overall carbohydrate limitation, with carbohydrate intake split into multiple small meals and snacks, also needs to be emphasized.

For blood glucose values above 200 mg/dl, urine ketone checks and close inspection of the pump and infusion site are needed, as well as changing the pump site after giving an injection by pen or syringe if the blood glucose is above 200–250 mg/dl.

Once the patient goes into labor, or is induced, the best way to handle the insulin pump will depend on the capabilities of the facility where the patient is expected to deliver. Some centers use IV insulin drips with glucose infusion during labor and delivery, in which case the pump would be discontinued until post-delivery. In other facilities where IV insulin protocols are not in place, or where the staff is familiar with and has protocols to guide the use of an insulin pump during labor, the pump should be continued. As is always the case for a pump patient in the hospital, the patient would need to have all her pump supplies necessary to change her infusion set and site readily available. There also needs to be a protocol in place to replace the need for insulin if the pump fails or the pump site dislodges and the patient is not able to replace it immediately. Active labor is exercise, during which the needs for insulin drop quickly, and the need for glucose rises rapidly (Jovanovic 2004). At a minimum, hourly monitoring of the blood glucose level is necessary during delivery.

One facility where insulin pumps (usually with CGM) are used extensively in pregnant pregestational diabetes is the East Virginia Medical Center in Norfolk, Virginia. (Marigrita de Veciana, MD, personal communication with Nicholas B. Argento, MD, November 2011). The facility has successfully implemented pump therapy into OB delivery. For elective inductions or C-sections, the patients are encouraged to change their pump site the day before the procedure. Patients on pumps are asked to sign an informed consent indicating that they understand they must supply all supplies for the pump, be capable of working and adjusting the pump themselves, and be willing to inform the staff of any changes in insulin therapy they make or boluses they take, and that, if their blood glucose is uncontrolled on the pump, they agree that they will be switched to an IV insulin drip per protocol. The pump patients are supplied with instructions on adjusting insulin rates if the diabetes-managing physician is not present, with a goal of keeping them between 80–120 mg/dl. For an elective C-section, generally the patients decrease the basal rate by 30% 8 hours before delivery, while NPO, or by 50% if they are hypoglycemia-prone. Patients admitted in labor or who are being induced will have their basal rates decreased by 30–50% once in labor, and are given D5-containing IV fluid. All patients have close and ongoing glucose monitoring. In the experience of the East Virginia Medical Center physicians, some but not most patients will come off insulin by the end of their labor, particularly those who had lower insulin needs to start with. These are general guidelines only, since the experience of individual patients can vary widely. Most patients are well controlled during delivery and are able to stay on their pump throughout their stay. If they cannot be well-controlled or are not able to work the pump, then IV insulin is started, if needed.

Post-delivery, the needs for insulin drop dramatically. Once the patient has delivered, her basal rates and insulin-to-carbohydrate bolus ratios should initially be reduced to 10–20% below those that she needed prepregnancy (if those rates and ratios are known), or reduced by 50% or more from the end-of-pregnancy rates and ratios if prepregnancy ratios are not known. Some type 1 patients may need little or no insulin for the first 12–24 hours post-delivery. The lower post-pregnancy rates should be written out toward the end of pregnancy and brought by the patient to the hospital. For patients who have a pump that allows multiple basal profiles, the lower basal profile could be entered during late pregnancy. Adjustments will be needed and close follow-up in this period is necessary. It is also important to emphasize to the patient that the target blood glucose levels need to be reset as well, to those appropriate for a non-pregnant adult, since it is not reasonable for most non-pregnant patients to try to maintain the very tight blood glucose goals necessary during pregnancy, which carry a high risk of hypoglycemia (Rosenn 1995).

# Pediatrics: Infants, Toddlers, Children, Teenagers

## Insulin Requirements in Children

Insulin pump use in infants and toddlers will likely increase with the ability of an insulin pump to deliver basal insulin rates of 0.01 to 0.025 units/hour (Bruttomesso 2009). During the "honeymoon period" and in infants and toddlers when insulin requirements are low, insulin in a pump can be diluted using a diluent, usually in a ratio of 1:10 (Wilson 2005; Bharucha 2005). Children are more insulin sensitive than adolescents, teenagers, and adults. When adjusting basal rates in children, incremental changes should be made in 10–15% increments, or 0.025 to 0.05 units/hour. Nocturnal hypoglycemia can be corrected by lowering the basal rate 2 to 3 hours before the occurrence of the hypoglycemic event. Children sometimes have a reverse dawn phenomenon requiring higher basal rates between 10:00 p.m. and 2:00 a.m. (ADA, Kaufman, 2012). It has been reported that prepubertal children have peak basal rates during the hours of 9 to 10 p.m., while children in puberty require higher basal doses in the early morning hours (Holterhus 2007). Some healthcare professionals prefer to implement lower basal rates at night for safety reasons, i.e., to prevent nocturnal hypoglycemia. Basal check tests (see "Basal Rate Adjustment" in Chapter 6) should be performed to fully assess the child's insulin requirements.

While current standards reflect the need to achieve and maintain glucose control to as nearnormogylcemia as safely possible, children have a unique risk for hypoglycemia. Research indicates that most children under the age of 6 or 7 have a form of "hypoglycemic unawareness," including immaturity of and a relative inability to recognize and respond to hypoglycemic symptoms, thus putting them at greater risk for severe hypoglycemia. Additionally, children under the age of 5 may be at risk for permanent cognitive impairment following episodes of severe hypoglycemia (ADA 2012; Asvold 2010; Northam 1998; Rovet 1997). And findings from the Diabetes Control and Complications Trial (DCCT) demonstrated that near-normalization of blood glucose levels was more difficult to achieve in adolescents than adults (DCCT Research Group 1993).

Due to the greater risk for hypoglycemia and difficulty in matching the ever-changing insulin needs in children, glycemic targets are set higher for children with diabetes (up to age 19) compared with adults with diabetes (American Diabetes Association, 2013) (Table 7).

## At What Age Is a Child Ready for a Pump?

Diabetes skills and knowledge vary according to developmental age (Table 8). Using an insulin pump can make diabetes management easier, but it can also create some challenges. There is no age recommendation for initiation of an insulin pump. Refer to the information below to help you decide if an insulin pump is right for your young patient. Additionally, consider the parents' as well as the young patient's readiness for insulin pump therapy.

## TABLE 7. Plasma Blood Glucose and A1C Goals for Type 1 Diabetes by Age Group

| Values by Age (years) | Plasma Blood Glucose Goal Range (mg/dl) | | A1C | Rationale |
|---|---|---|---|---|
| | Before Meals | Bedtime/ Overnight | | |
| Toddlers and preschoolers (0–6) | 100–180 | 110–200 | <8.5% | • Vulnerability to hypoglycemia<br>• Insulin sensitivity<br>• Unpredictability in dietary intake and physical activity<br>• A lower goal (<8.0%) is reasonable if it can be achieved without excessive hypoglycemia |
| School age (6–12) | 90–180 | 100–180 | <8% | • Vulnerability to hypoglycemia<br>• A lower goal (<7.5%) is reasonable if it can be achieved without excessive hypoglycemia |
| Adolescents and young adults (13–19) | 90–130 | 90–150 | <7.5% | • A lower goal (<7.0%) is reasonable if it can be achieved without excessive hypoglycemia |

**Key concepts in setting glycemic goals:**
- Goals should be individualized and lower goals may be reasonable based on benefit–risk assessment.
- Blood glucose goals should be modified in children with frequent hypoglycemia or hypoglycemia unawareness.
- Postprandial blood glucose values should be measured when there is a discrepancy between preprandial blood glucose values and A1C levels and to help assess glycemia in those on basal/bolus regimens.

## TABLE 8. Diabetes and Insulin Pump Knowledge and Skills by Developmental Age

| Age | Knowledge | Skills |
|---|---|---|
| Birth to age 3; infants and toddlers | Inherent trust in parents/caregivers | Rapid changes in cognitive and motor skills, nutrition requirements, sleep/wake patterns, and acquisition of developmental milestones<br>Concerns with pump placement, skin, infusion sites, tubing<br>Parents/caregivers perform all tasks |
| 3–5 years, preschool | Aware of presence of pump<br>Begin to ask about food items and if they can be consumed and require a bolus<br>More interactive with peers who are interested in the pump | Lacks motor skills and cognitive ability to contribute to diabetes management<br>Interact with decisions regarding placement of infusion set and pump |
| 6–9 years, school-aged | Continued reliance on parents/caregiver for diabetes decisions<br>Minimally explain diabetes and has increasing awareness of tasks and goals<br>Understand importance of blood glucose control and glucose numbers<br>Understand that exercise can cause hypoglycemia<br>Ask about food<br>May feel different from peers<br>May begin to feel self-conscious about diabetes | Wear pump appropriately<br>Help insert pump infusion set<br>Disconnect pump to give to supervising adult<br>Be responsible for pump when disconnected<br>Reconnect pump with assistance<br>Activate bolus dose with direction |
| 10–12 years | Count carbohydrate<br>Begin to calculate insulin dose for meals and corrections using pump's bolus calculator feature<br>Understand diabetes management goals<br>Understand exercise can cause hypoglycemia | Protect infusion site<br>Protect pump during activity<br>Disconnect and reconnect pump<br>Insert infusion set<br>Activate bolus dose |

*(Table continues on next page)*

| TABLE 8. Diabetes and Insulin Pump Knowledge and Skills by Developmental Age *(Continued)* | | |
|---|---|---|
| **Age** | **Knowledge** | **Skills** |
| 13–14 years | Calculate and deliver bolus Understand the role of exercise Recognize need for basal rate changes Issues with image and body weight Self-conscious about pump Rebellion and risk-taking behavior | Significant increase in insulin requirements Erratic eating and sleeping behaviors Forgets meal and correction boluses Can manage most tasks, but may need assistance with bolus calculation and programming/changing basal rates Suspend/stop basal delivery |
| 15–18 years | Increased independence, parental conflict Determine factors that affect basal rates and how to perform basal check tests Determine changes in basal rates, with assistance Determine factors that affect bolus doses Change insulin-to-carbohydrate ratio(s) (ICR) and correction/sensitivity factor(s) (CF) Use sick-day guidelines, with guidance | Program changes in basal rates Program changes in ICR and CF |

(Adapted from: Kaufman 2012; Bode 2012)

Considerations for pump therapy in the pediatric patient include:

1. Recurrent severe hypoglycemia
2. Wide fluctuations in blood glucose levels, regardless of A1C level
3. Inflexible insulin regimen that achieves target glucose levels but is difficult to fit into lifestyle

4. A1C level above target
5. Ketosis-prone
6. Microvascular complications and/or risk factors for macrovascular complications
7. Eating disorder
8. Needle phobia
9. Pregnancy
10. Competitive athlete
    (Philip 2007)

Pump therapy success in the youth requires that the child or adolescent is receptive to pump therapy (depending on age and maturity) and has strong family support. Evidence indicates that the use of insulin pumps in children ranging from infancy to adolescence in families in which parents and children together manage the child's diabetes can result in achievement of ADA glucose targets (Nimri 1997; Doyle 2004). Insulin pump therapy in children has a positive effect on quality of life (Batajoo 2012).

A strong commitment and motivation on the part of both parents and child to master the basics of pump therapy during the learning curve is a must in order for the child to succeed with his/her pump. Parents must have a thorough understanding of what an insulin pump can and cannot do and be willing to take on the additional learning that pump therapy requires. No matter what the age, diabetes management can be challenging and overwhelming. And although there is no age that is "too young" or "right" for pump therapy initiation, explain realistic expectations and the parents' role and responsibilities when discussing pump therapy for a young child; pump therapy may not be appropriate for every young child. Discontinuation rates of insulin pump therapy in children range from 7 to 18% and may be attributed to the strict criteria for treatment initiation imposed by pediatric centers (Maahs 2010), but ultimately, the decision to choose pump therapy for a child should be individualized with the guidance from the child's multidisciplinary diabetes management team (Fuld 2010; Philip 2007). Additionally, pump therapy initiation in a child should be based on the decision of the child's HCP and parents/caregiver, not on the insurance company (Eugster 2006), although coverage of insulin pump supplies after the child reaches the age (26 as of this writing) when s/he is no longer insured by their parents' insurance company may be a factor to keep in mind.

The same basic guidelines for adults who use a pump are also pertinent for children—i.e., regarding infusion sets, pump settings and the "buttonology," wearing the pump, etc. Advise parents to take advantage of commercial products available for wearing a pump—the Internet is a good place to start (see Chapter 8, Forms and Resources). There are many child–and young adult–specific items. Remind parents that although most adults can be disconnected from their pump for a maximum of 2 hours, 1 hour is the maximum recommended for children.

## Young Children: Infants, Toddlers, and Pre-school Children

Insulin pump therapy use in babies, toddlers, and pre-school children is becoming increasingly popular (Hofer 2012). Pediatric patients are often impulsive, finicky eaters and can be unpredictable in their amount and duration of physical activity. And children with diabetes are insulin sensitive and can experience erratic blood glucose levels with bouts of frequent or severe hypoglycemia and hyperglycemia. An insulin pump can be a useful tool to help establish and fine-tune control. And as parents and caretakers struggle with achieving and maintaining glucose control in their child, the use of this technology can offer hope to assist in this challenge.

**Advantages of Pump Therapy for Young Children**
- Flexibility and freedom in schedule, meal timing
- Fewer injections
- Increased convenience compared with insulin pen or syringe preparation and injections
- Personalization of 24=h basal dosing, especially during growth spurts
- Establishment of appropriate basal insulin for the dawn phenomenon
- Absence of long-duration basal insulin following unplanned exercise/activity

- Individualization of meal/snack dosing for erratic or unplanned (carbohydrate) intake
- Precise dosing in small increments/units for meals, snacks, and hyperglycemia
- Bolus calculators
- Insulin-on-board information
- Ease in adjusting basal insulin for exercise and sports
- Ease in adjusting insulin doses during travel
- Less hypoglycemia (nocturnal as well as daytime)
- "Fitting in" with other young children during special events (e.g., parties, sleepovers)
- Data storage, e.g., history of insulin doses, carbohydrate intake, etc.
- Improved quality of life
- Long-term glucose control that can delay or prevent onset of complications

## Disadvantages of Pump Therapy for Young Children

- Psychological concerns
- 24–h attachment to a device
- Wearing/attachment concerns and challenges
- Fear and pain of infusion set or patch pump insertion
- Skin irritation
- Tape removal
- Risk of infection
- Displacement, accidental or intentional removal during playtime, naps, and sleep
- Unavailability of supplies following infusion set change or empty cartridge/reservoir
- Caretaker unfamiliarity with pump in response to alert/alarm or problem
- Risk of diabetic ketoacidosis (DKA) following disconnection from pump

- Risk of hypoglycemia from incorrect doses (basal, bolus) or "stacking" of bolus doses
- Frequent SMBG
- Repeated basal rate testing, especially during growth spurts
- Forgotten meal boluses (unless pump alarms are set)
- Potential for weight gain
- Learning curve for the parents and caretaker(s)
- Expense

## Parents' Roles and Responsibilities

When pump therapy is initiated in an infant, toddler, or young child, it is the parents who must be educated by the healthcare professional team (physician/ diabetes educator[s]) and trained by the pump manufacturer trainer in the button-pushing aspects of the pump. Likewise, the parents need to assume the responsibilities normally relegated to the adult pump wearer, including knowledge of carbohydrate counting and the child's insulin-to-carbohydrate ratio(s), correction (sensitivity) factors, duration of insulin action (similar to that of adults), and target blood glucose levels.

Basal doses in young children may be as low as 0.025 units per hour, and bolus doses can be as low as 0.05 units. Advise parents to compare pump models carefully to choose the pump best suited for their child's needs. Some pumps offer tamper-resistant or "lock-out" features for settings—this can be helpful when using the pump in a young child.

Children today are exposed to technology at a very young age, and a child as young as 4 or 5, depending on their maturity and cognitive ability, may be able to program their pump. However, caution parents that knowing how to press buttons is different from knowing and understanding the reasons for pushing buttons in a specific sequence. Parents need to provide direct supervision for their child's pump until approximately age 8 because most children under that age lack the cognitive skills to program their pump. At about age 8 to 9, children can be taught to program their own boluses. And until age 9–10, an infusion set insertion is the parents' responsibility. The tubing of an infusion set used by a child can be a shorter length, and an extra piece of tape or dressing can help anchor the pump's tubing to the skin. A tubeless or patch pump may be a good option to consider.

Bolus insulin doses should be based on carbohydrate counting to assure success with an insulin pump (Waldron 2002). Children of all ages tend to snack, thus require more frequent bolus doses than adults who may eat just two to three times per day. Research reveals that bolus doses in excess of 7 per day have been associated with lower A1C levels (Danne 2005). As an alternative to an increased number of injections with multiple daily injection (MDI) therapy, an insulin pump is an attractive option.

The timing of bolus doses may need to be adjusted, as boluses may be best given following completion of a meal or snack versus preprandially, as the child's intake is often impulsive, unpredictable, and erratic. When given postprandially, the bolus insulin dose can better match what the child has actually eaten (Rutledge 1997). Use of the pump's bolus reminder alert setting for a missed meal bolus will help alleviate a forgotten bolus. And, use of the pump's extended and combination bolus features will be beneficial for the child who enjoys the occasional high-fat (fast) food and pizza (Refer to Chapter 7, Dining Out and Special Meals: Bolus Options). Frequent blood glucose monitoring is another important responsibility of the parents, either as caregivers performing the blood glucose checks, or in a "supervisory" role for the older child's SMBG.

## The School-Aged Child

Similarly to the very young child, the school-aged child must have supportive parents in order to be successful with insulin pump therapy. Additionally, the child's school personnel must learn and understand the basics of diabetes as well as the basics of insulin pump therapy. Parents must become familiar with school regulations and establish positive communication through meetings and a written diabetes management plan. Advise parents of their rights under the Americans with Disabilities Act and the importance of working with the child's teacher(s) and school nurse (and other school personnel as needed) to create a plan that allows their child to be effectively and safely managed in school (Kaufman 2012). It is challenging for school personnel to understand diabetes, and insulin pump therapy can be an additional hurdle for them to comprehend.

Parents must devise three management plans for their child. The plans clearly outline what is required for success with diabetes management and insulin pump therapy:

1. Diabetes Medical Management Plan (DMMP): completed by the child's healthcare team; contains the medical orders that are the basis for the child's healthcare and education plan
2. Individualized Health Plan (IHP): developed by the school nurse in collaboration with the child's healthcare team and family; serves to implement the medical recommendations in the student's DMMP into use at the school
3. Emergency care plan for the treatment of hypoglycemia and hyperglycemia: based on the medical orders; provides guidance on how to recognize and treat hypoglycemia and hyperglycemia and includes contact names for assistance; developed by the school nurse and should be distributed to all school personnel who are responsible for the child with diabetes during the school day and after-school activities (Kaufman 2012)

The DMMP should contain information about the child's diabetes, including details about the insulin pump (brand, model, serial number, and who to contact for pump problems). It is beyond the scope of this book to provide inclusive DMMP information. Refer parents to become familiar with the federal laws that address the school's responsibilities to assist the child with diabetes: (1) Section 504 of the Rehabilitation Act of 1973; (2) the Americans with Disabilities Act (ADA) of 1990; and (3) the Individuals with Disabilities Education Act (IDEA). The American Diabetes Association also has the "Safe at School" program to assist parents of school-aged children with diabetes (ADA 2012).

When working with parents of a child using an insulin pump, consider the who, what, where, and when: who will count the carbohydrate in the child's snack or meal and determine the correct bolus dose?; what will be done in the classroom versus the nurse's office; what backup supplies are necessary (refer to "Emergency Supplies" in Chapter 6)?; where will the child perform SMBG or obtain blood glucose checks and deliver bolus doses?; when will blood glucose checks and bolus doses be administered? The ability to perform routine blood glucose checks (by meter or CGM) in the classroom, cafeteria, gymnasium, or elsewhere becomes a normal part of the day and the child with diabetes as well as other children can view the task as routine (Kaufman 2012).

It is crucial that school personnel understand that the child's insulin pump must not be removed and a dislodged infusion set or patch pod must be replaced immediately. A child with diabetes wearing an insulin pump should be encouraged to participate in school activities, including field trips and physical education ("gym"). The child's classmates will be curious about the insulin pump and may ask to touch it to see how it works. The child should be aware of any buttons that might be pushed during such times and what s/he needs to do in such a situation. Appropriate supervision for diabetes management, including the pump, is essential.

## Babysitters and Day Care

Entrusting your child to others can create anxiety for the child as well as for the parents. Advise parents to prepare their child's babysitter and day care personnel with the basics about your child's diabetes and insulin pump therapy. Parents should provide detailed instructions for handling routine tasks, such as feeding the child, as well as what to do and who to contact in case of an emergency. The parents, if comfortable having the babysitter or daycare personnel perform this task, must provide insulin pump button-pushing training for the delivery of any necessary bolus insulin.

## Adolescents and Teenagers

During adolescence, growth spurts will necessitate changes in insulin doses, most notably with the onset of a pattern of unexplainable hyperglycemia. The onset of puberty increases insulin requirements. Be aware of the need to perform more frequent basal checks to determine appropriate basal rate changes. Additionally, the insulin-to-carbohydrate ratio(s) and correction/sensitivity factor(s) may also need to be adjusted (refer to "Basal Rate Adjustment, Insulin-to-Carbohydrate Ratio Adjustment; and Correction (Sensitivity) Factor Adjustment" in Chapter 6).

Insulin pump use during adolescence in children with type 1 diabetes has been reported to be safe and effective (Plotnick 2003; Daane 2008). However, retrospective research indicates diabetic ketoacidosis in this age-group can occur due to pump malfunction and infusion site inflammation (Cope 2008), although that is also true with pump use in any age-group. Parental involvement can have a positive impact on the child's A1C level (Plotnick 2003) while reducing the risk of severe hypoglycemia and enhancing diabetes management coping skills (Boland 1999).

The teenage years can be turbulent for any parents, but for the parents of a teenager with diabetes, the challenges can be multi-fold. During this time, teenagers begin to exert their independence and may find managing their diabetes is burdensome and "gets in the way." Pump therapy may be an appealing option for the teen who is complaining of "having to watch the clock," taking frequent injections, and experiencing a pattern of extreme highs and lows. "Sleeping in" on weekends is easier with a pump, i.e., the basal rate will continue to provide the necessary insulin to achieve target glucose levels. This is also true for "sleepovers" for children of all ages, assuming the nocturnal basal rate(s) is correct. Psychological support is helpful and reinforcement of both parent and adolescent/teenager responsibilities is paramount. Pump use in this age group requires ongoing communication and clear role delineation among the pumper, parents, and clinician. And pump therapy use during the college years will help manage hectic schedules, stress, fast food, and sports. When considering a pump, point out the advantages for lifestyle flexibility, but also reinforce the importance of the time investment in training, pump initiation, and frequent communication with the HCP and/or diabetes team to assure success.

# Type 2 and Type 1.5 (LADA) Diabetes

Insulin pump therapy in patients with type 2 diabetes has been used for many years. Studies show that patients with type 2 diabetes in suboptimal control using oral agents achieve better control with pump therapy (Ilkova 1997; Valensi 1997). Large clinical studies in insulin-using patients with type 2 diabetes demonstrated that pump therapy resulted in control similar to that of MDI regimens, while smaller studies revealed that pump therapy was superior to MDI therapy (Bode 2010). A clinical trial examining the short-term (2–3 weeks) use of pump therapy in newly diagnosed patients with type 2 diabetes showed that pump therapy resulted in improvements in glycemic control, $\beta$-cell function, and insulin sensitivity that resulted in long-term remission without anti-diabetes medication. The pump therapy patients also achieved higher scores in positive attitude and self-care behavior and ability compared with patients who experienced relapse (Chen 2012). And although the clinical evidence to support widespread use is mixed, pump therapy in type 2 diabetes is a promising option for those patients who require MDI therapy. A pump may be an appealing option to a patient with type 2 diabetes who has needle phobia or suffers from (or has fear of) difficult-to-manage frequent or nocturnal hypoglycemia. And the use of U-500 insulin in an insulin pump in a highly insulin-resistant patient with type 2 diabetes, although not yet FDA-approved, is growing and may be an attractive option to improve diabetes control and management (refer to "Additional Considerations" and "Use of U-500 Human Regular Insulin in an Insulin Pump" in Chapter 5).

Insurance coverage of pump therapy in type 2 diabetes and LADA is a concern. Make sure you and your potential pump patient are aware of your patient's insurance coverage, e.g., Medicare or supplemental coverage, prior to proceeding with the pump order/initiation process. As of this writing, Medicare provides coverage for an insulin pump in patients whose C-peptide or the beta cell autoantibody test meets Medicare's definition of diabetes (DHHS 2013). Refer to "Profile of an Appropriate Candidate" and "A Good Prospect: Ready, Willing, and Able" in Chapter 3 for additional information on Medicare coverage.

Use the same criteria for evaluating a pump candidate with type 2/LADA diabetes as you would use for a patient or parents of a child with type 1 diabetes.

Pump therapy in patients with type 2 diabetes may be beneficial for those with:

- needle phobia during MDI therapy
- erratic use of injection regimen, i.e. frequently missed or omitted MDI doses
- concerns about "chasing insulin," i.e., eating excess or unwanted calories to prevent hypoglycemia
- continued weight gain as a result of insulin therapy, perhaps from "chasing insulin"
- frequent hypoglycemia
- nocturnal hypoglycemia
- substantial dawn phenomenon
- erratic lifestyle and struggling with MDI therapy
- fairly routine or standard eating patterns
- pregnancy
- insulin resistance or already using U-500 insulin syringe therapy (and willing to do the "conversion" factor calculations using U-500 insulin in a pump)

■ an adequate support system, e.g., do not live alone
■ confirmed insurance- or self-pay coverage of the pump supplies

Pump therapy is contraindicated in patients with type 2 diabetes who have:

■ high (>150 units) daily insulin requirements, as pump cartridges/ reservoirs volume maximum may be about 300 units, thus requiring frequent (daily or every-other-day cartridge/reservoir refills)
■ technology challenges or concerns
■ cognitive impairment
■ an inadequate support system, i.e., lives alone
■ low or fixed income and may not be able to afford the pump supplies
■ decreased or impaired vision without adequate support
■ decreased hearing or hearing loss without adequate support
■ diminished dexterity without adequate support

Pump initiation in patients with type 2 or type 1.5 diabetes is the same as in type 1 diabetes. Refer to Chapter 5, Pump Start-Up, for pump start guidelines. Many clinicians use weight to calculate a starting Total Daily Dose (TDD): 0.5 × kg/body weight OR 0.24/lb/body weight = the starting TDD. Divide the TDD equally, 50% for basal needs, and 50% for boluses, and divide the bolus total between the number of meals the person eats. Keep in mind that many patients with type 2 diabetes consume only two major meals/day (breakfast and a late afternoon lunch/dinner combination meal), with a snack in the evening.

A bolus option calculation for people with type 2 or type 1.5 diabetes may be determined by a smart pump feature that calculates the meal dose based on settings entered during pump initiation/setup. This method uses an amount of insulin per meal based on a fixed or set amount of grams of carbohydrate (or "average/usual" amount) the person consumes/enters into the pump (here's where a registered dietitian (RD) CDE prepump initiation would be most helpful in determining the amount of carbohydrate the person consumes). For patients who are not adept at or comfortable using carb counting, this method of using a "fixed" amount of carb/meal used to calculate the premeal insulin may be useful. Ideally, of course, carb counting would be more accurate, but for a patient whose meal intake is typically standard day to day and without great variation in carbohydrate amounts, this "simple" method may be useful. The use of a simple insulin dosing regimen in a pump-using patient with type 2 diabetes has been shown to improve glycemic control without severe hypoglycemia with limited weight gain (Edelman 2010).

Prior to determining the insulin dose, the patient must know the number of carbohydrate grams s/he consumes for each "type" of meal, e.g., snack, small meal, medium-sized meal, large meal. Instead of using or learning carb counting, which, of course, is more specific, the patient uses a "standard" amount of carb usually consumed at the type of meal they eat. Again, an RD or CDE can be consulted to help the patient determine these amounts.

1. Using the 450 or 500 Rule (see "Pump Start-Up, Calculating Insulin-to-Carbohydrate Ratios [ICR]" in Chapter 5), calculate the patient's ICR.
2. During the initial pump setup, the ICR(s) would be entered into the pump's settings.
3. Review with the patient the number of grams of carbohydrate to enter for the type of meal about to be consumed (ideally calculated/determined by the RD, CDE), e.g., snack = 30 g; small = 45 ± 5 g; medium = 60 ± 5 g; large = 75 ± 5 g.
4. Following the steps for the particular pump, the patient will enter their current blood glucose level and the number of grams of carbohydrate to be consumed.
5. The pump's "bolus calculator" feature will automatically calculate the recommended dose of insulin.

## Medication Adjustments for Patients with Type 2 or LADA/Type 1.5 Diabetes

Upon initiation of insulin pump therapy in a patient with type 2 or type 1.5 diabetes, stop medication that directly affects insulin secretion. These include sulfonylureas (such as glyburide, glipizide, glimepiride) and meglitinides (repaglinide, nateglinide). Non-insulin hormonal system medications such as a biguanide (metformin), amylin analog (pramlintide), alpha-glucosidase inhibitor, incretin mimetic, or insulin sensitizer (thiazolidinedione) may be continued per FDA-approved use with a rapid-acting insulin analog.

In patients with insulin resistance, improvements in blood glucose may necessitate a reduction in total daily doses of insulin, thus necessitating changes in basal rates, ICR(s), and CF(s).

## Pump Use in Type 2 Diabetes and Pregnancy

A study conducted in Australia in patients with gestational diabetes or type 2 diabetes and pregnancy with ongoing hyperglycemia requiring a maximum insulin dose of 100 to 199 units/day revealed that 79% of the women experienced improved glycemic control within 1 to 4 weeks after pump therapy initiation (Simmons 2001). The pump patients had greater weight gain and an increase in insulin requirements, and none reported severe hypoglycemia. Infants born to pump-using patients with type 2 diabetes in this study were more likely to be admitted to the special care baby unit, but were not likely to experience greater hypoglycemia and were not heavier than control patients' babies. Pump therapy use in type 2 diabetes and pregnancy can be considered a safe option to improve glycemic control in those patients who require large doses of insulin.

# Older Adults and Special Needs Patients

The American Geriatrics Society recommends that older adults (those >60 years of age) who are able to perform self-care, self-maintenance, and physical activities should strive to maintain glycemic goals consistent with ADA standards (Brown 2003). Based on expert consensus or clinical experience, the ADA *Standards of Medical Care in Diabetes—2013* states that insulin use requires patients or caregivers have good visual and motor skills and cognitive ability. Furthermore, patients who can be expected to live long enough to benefit from long-term intensive diabetes management and who are active, have good cognitive function, and are willing to learn and apply their skills should be provided with the needed education and skills to do so and be treated using the goals for younger adults with diabetes (ADA 2013). Presently, more than 25% of the U.S. population aged ≥65 years has diabetes (Centers for Disease Control and Prevention 2011; Kirkman 2012). There are few long-term studies in older adults with diabetes demonstrating the benefits of intensive therapy and even fewer studies using insulin pumps in older adults. The risk of hypoglycemia must be considered in considering insulin (and thus, pump) therapy in older adults. Keep in mind the factors presented above (in type 2 diabetes) when considering pump therapy in an older patient. Although the data are limited, pump therapy can be successful. In otherwise healthy and functional older adults (mean age

66 years), pump or MDI therapy use resulted in a mean A1C of 7% that was able to be maintained for 12 months with low rates of hypoglycemia (Herman 2005).

Some older patients or patients with special needs include those with:

- decreased or impaired vision
- decreased hearing or hearing loss
- diminished manual dexterity
- impaired or limited cognitive ability

Today's pumps offer brighter, larger, lighted screens with color or touch ability. Some pumps are more or less sophisticated than others, and there may be a pump model that is especially appealing to those patients with certain challenges or needs. Pump functions can be audio and some brands offer selections in several volume choices. Use of a "touch" bolus button with either vibration or sound, or both, is another option available to those with vision or hearing challenges. The special needs patient who expresses interest in or is receptive to insulin pump therapy should be made aware of the various brands and options. Pump models are constantly improving with better, more user-friendly technology. Make sure you are up-to-date with your knowledge of the latest and greatest pump models so that you can inform your patient of pumps that might have otherwise not been available several months earlier (refer to Chapter 8, Forms and Resources).

## REFERENCES

AccuChek Insulin Pumps: https://www.accu-chek.com/us/# Accessed 10 February 2013

American Diabetes Association: 2013 clinical practice recommendations. *Diabetes Care* 36 (Suppl. 1):S11–S66, 2013

American Diabetes Association, Kaufman FR, ed.: *Medical Management of Type 1 Diabetes,* 6th ed., Alexandria, VA: American Diabetes Association, 2012

American Diabetes Association: *Fact Sheet—Air Travel and Diabetes.* http://www.diabetes.org/assets/pdfs/know-your-rights/public-accommodations/air-travel-and-diabetes.pdf Accessed 10 February 2013

American Diabetes Association: Nutrition recommendations and interventions for diabetes (Position Statement). *Diabetes Care* 31 (Suppl. 1):S61–S78, 2008

American Diabetes Association: Physical activity/exercise and diabetes (Position Statement). *Diabetes Care* 27 (Suppl. 1):S58–S62, 2004

American Diabetes Association: *Safe at School* http://www.diabetes.org/living-with-diabetes/parents-and-kids/diabetes-care-at-school/ Accessed 10 February 2013

Animas Insulin Pumps: http://www.animas.com/faq/other-airport-security Accessed 10 February 2013

Arky RA, Veverbrand E, Abramson EA: Irreversible hypoglycemia: a complication of alcohol and insulin. *JAMA* 206:575–578, 1968

Asvold BO, Sand T, Hestad K, Bjørgaas MR: Cognitive function in type 1 diabetic adults with early exposure to severe hypoglycemia: a 16-year follow-up study. *Diabetes Care* 33:1945–1947, 2010

Batajoo RJ, Messina CR, Wilson TA: Long-term efficacy of insulin pump therapy in children with type 1 diabetes mellitus. *J Clin Res Pediatr Endocrinol* 4:127–131, 2012

Bharucha T, Brown J, McDonnell C, Gebert R, McDougall P, Cameron F, Werther G, Zacharin M: Neonatal diabetes mellitus: insulin pump as an alternative management strategy. *J Paediatr Child Health* 41:522–526, 2005

Ben G, Gnidi L, Maran A, Gigante A, Duner E, Iori E, Tiengo A, Avogaro A: Effects of chronic alcohol intake on carbohydrate and lipid metabolism in subjects with type II (non-insulin-ependent) diabetes. *Am J Med* 90:70–76, 1991

Bode BW, Kyllo J, Kaufman FR: *Medtronic Pumping Protocol: A Guide to Insulin Pump Therapy Initiation.* Northridge, CA: Medtronic, Inc./Diabetes, 2012

Bode BW: Insulin pump use in type 2 diabetes. *Diabetes Technol Ther* 12 (Suppl. 1):S17–21, 2010

Boland EA, Grey M, Oesterle A, Fredridkson L, Tamborlane WV: Continuous subcutaneous insulin infusion. A new way to lower risk of severe hypoglycemia, improve metabolic control, and enhance cooping in adolescents with type 1 diabetes. *Diabetes Care* 22:1179–1184, 1999

Brown AF, Mangione DM, Saliba D, Sarkisian CA; California Healthcare Foundation/American Geriatrics Society Panel on Improving Care for Elders With Diabetes: Guidelines for improving the care of the older person with diabetes mellitus. *J Am Geriatr Soc* 51 (Suppl Guidelines):S265-S280, 2003.

Burdick J, Chase HP, Slover RH, Knievel K, Scrimgeour L, Maniatis AK, Klingensmith GJ: Missed insulin meal boluses and elevated hemoglobin A1c levels in children receiving insulin pump therapy. *Pediatrics* 113:221–224, 2004

Centers for Disease Control and Prevention: *National Diabetes Fact Sheet: General Information and National Estimates on Diabetes in the United States, 2011.* Atlanta, GA, U.S. Department of Health and Human Services, Centers for Disease Control and Prevention, 2011

Chase HP, Saib SZ, MacKenzie T, Hansen MM, and Garg SK: Postprandial glucose excursions following four methods of bolus insulin administration in subjects with type 1 diabetes. *Diabet Med* 19:317–21, 2002

Chen A, Huyang Z, Wan X, Deng W, Wu J, Li L, Cai Q, Xiao H, LI Y: Attitudes toward diabetes affect maintenance of drug-free remission in patients with newly diagnosed type 2 diabetes after short-term continuous subcutaneous insulin infusion treatment. *Diabetes Care* 35:474–481, 2012

Cobry E, McFann K, Messer L, Gage V, VanderWel B, Horton L, Chase HP: Timing of meal boluses to achieve optimal postprandial glycemic control in patients with type 1 diabetes. *Diabetes Technol Ther* 12:173–177, 2010

Cope JU, Morrison AE, Samuels-Reid J: Adolescent use of insulin and patient-controlled analgesia pump technology: a 10-year Food and Drug Administration retrospective study of adverse events. *Pediatrics* 121:e1133–1138, 2008

Coyle E: Fluid and carbohydrate replacement during exercise: how much and why? *Sports Science Exchange* 7:1–6, 1994

Danne T, Battelino T, Jarosz-Chobot P, Kordonouri O, Pánkowska E, Ludvigsson J, Schober E, Kaprio E, Saukkonen T, Nicolino M, Tubiana-Rufi N, Klinkert C, Haberland H, Vazeou A, Madacsy L, Zangen D, Cherubini V, Rabbone I, Toni S, de Beaufort C, Bakker-van Waarde W, van den Berg N, Volkov I, Barrio R, Hanas R, Zumsteg U, Kuhlmann B, Aebi C, Schumacher U, Gschwend S, Hindmarsh P, Torres M, Shehadeh N, Phillip M; PedPump Study Group: Establishing glycaemic control with continuous subcutaneous insulin infusion in children and adolescents with type 1 diabetes: experience of the PedPump study in 17 countries. *Diabetologia* 51:1594–1601, 2008

Danne T, Battelino T, Jarosz-Chobot P, Kordonouri O, Pánkowska E, Philip M, the PedPump Study Group: The PedPump Study: a low percentage of basal insulin and more than five boluses are associated with better centralized HbA1c in 1041 children on CSII from 17 countries (Abstract). *Diabetes* 54 (Suppl. 1):A453, 2005

Delahanty L, Simkins SW, Camelon K: Expanded role of the dietician in the Diabetes Control and Complications Trial: implications for clinical practice. The DCCT Research Group. *J Am Diet Assoc* 93:758–767, 1993

Department of Health and Human Services (DHHS) Centers for Medicare and Medicaid Services: National Coverage Determination (NCD) for Infusion PUMPs (280.14) http://www.cms.gov/medicare-coverage-database/details/nca-details.aspx?NCAId=40&NcaName=Insulin+Infusion+Pump&CoverageSelection=National&KeyWord=insulin+pump&KeyWordlookUp=Title&KeyWordSearchType=And&bc=gAAAABAAAAAA& Accessed 10 February 2013

Dexcom: www.dexcom.com Accessed 10 February 2013

Diabetes Control and Complications Trial Research Group: The effect of intensive treatment of diabetes on the development and progression of long-term complications in insulin-dependent diabetes mellitus. *N Engl J Med* 329:977–986, 1993

DirectNet Study Group: Prevention of hypoglycemia during exercise in children with type 1 diabetes by suspending basal insulin. *Diabetes Care* 29:2200–2204, 2006

Doyle EA, Weinzimer SA, Steffen AT, Ahern JA, Vincent M, Tamborlane WV: A randomized, prospective trial comparing the efficacy of continuous subcutaneous insulin infusion with multiple daily injections using insulin glargine. *Diabetes Care* 27:1554–1558, 2004

Edelman SV, Bode BW, Bailey TS, Kipnes MS, Brunelle R, Chen X, Frias JP: Insulin pump therapy in patients with type 2 diabetes safely improved glycemic control using a simple insulin dosing regimen. *Diabetes Technol Ther* 12:627–632, 2010

Eli Lilly and Company: *Humalog (insulin lispro injection USP [rDNA origin]) for Injection Prescribing Information.* Indianapolis, IN: Eli Lilly and Company, 2011

Eugster EA, Francis G, Lawson-Wilkins Drug and Therapeutics Committee: Position statement: continuous subcutaneous insulin infusion in very young children with type 1 diabetes. *Pediatrics* 118:e1244–1249, 2006

Feingold KR, Siperstein MD: Normalization of fasting blood glucose levels in insulin-requiring diabetes: the role of ethanol abstention. *Diabetes Care* 6:186–188, 1983

Franz MJ: Protein controversies in diabetes. *Diabetes Spectrum* 13:132, 2000

Franz MJ, Bantle JP, Beebe CA, Brunzell JD, Chiasson JL, Garg A, Holzmeister LA, Hoogwerf B, Mayer-Davis E, Mooradian AD, Purnell JQ, Wheeler M: Evidence-based nutrition principles and recommendations for the treatment and prevention of diabetes and related complications. *Diabetes Care* 25:148–198, 2002

Frezza M, di Padova C, Pozzato G, Terpin M, Baraona E, Lieber CS: High blood alcohol levels in women. The role of decreased gastric alcohol dehydrogenase activity and first-pass metabolism. *N Engl J Med* 322:95–99, 1990

Frohnauer MK, Liu K, Devlin JT: Adjustment of basal lispro insulin in CSII to minimize glycemic fluctuations caused by exercise. *Diab Res Clin Pract* 50 (Suppl. 1):S80, 2000

Fuld K, Conrad B, Buckingham B, Wilson DM: Insulin pumps in young children. *Diab Technol Ther* 12 (Suppl. 1):S67–S71, 2010

Gannon MC, Nuttall JA, Damberg G, Gupta V, Nuttall FQ: Effect of protein ingestion on the glucose appearance rate in people with type 2 diabetes. *J Clin Endocrinol Metab* 86:1040–1047, 2001

Gross RM, Kayne D, King A, Rother C, Juth S: A bolus calculator is an effective means of controlling postprandial glycemia in patients on insulin pump therapy. *Diabetes Technol Ther* 5:365–369, 2003

Grunberger G, Bailey TS, Cohen AJ, Flood TM, Handelsman Y, Hellman R, Jovanovic L, Moghissi ES, Orzeck EA: AACE insulin pump management task force statement by the American Association of Clinical Endocrinologists consensus panel on insulin pump management. *Endocr Pract* 16:746–762, 2010

Herman WH, Ilag LL, Johnson SL, Martin CL, Sinding J, Al Harthi A, Plunkett CD, LaPorte FB, Burke R, Brown MB, Halter JB, Raskin P: A clinical trial of continuous subcutaneous insulin infusion versus multiple daily injections in older adults with type 2 diabetes. *Diabetes Care* 28:1568–1573, 2005

Hirsch IB: Hitting the dartboard from 40,000 feet. *Diabetes Technol Therap* 13:981–982, 2011

Hirsch IB: Practical pearls in insulin pump therapy. *Diabetes Technol Therap* 12 (Suppl. 1):S23–S27, 2010

Hirsch IB: Insulin analogues. *N Engl J Med* 352:174–183, 2005

Hofer S, Meraner D, Koehle J: Insulin pump treatment in children and adolescents with type 1 diabetes. *Minerva Pediatr* 64:433–448, 2012

Holterhus PM, Odendahl R, Oesingmann S, Lepler R, Wagner V, Hiort O, Holl R: Classification of distinct baseline insulin infusion patterns in children and adolescents with type 1 diabetes on continuous subcutaneous insulin infusion therapy. *Diabetes Care* 30:568–573, 2007

Ilkova H, Galser B, Tunckale A, Bagriacik N, Cerasi E: Induction of long-term glycemic control in newly diagnosed type 2 diabetic patients by transient intensive insulin treatment. *Diabetes Care* 20:1353–1356, 1997

Ismail K, Winkley K, Rabe-Hesketh S: Systemic review and meta-analysis of randomized controlled trials of psychological interventions to improve glycaemic control in patients with type 2 diabetes. *Lancet* 363:1589–1597, 2004

Jones SM, Quarry JL, Caldwell-McMillan M, Mauger D, Gabbay R: Optimal insulin pump dosing and postprandial glycemia following a pizza meal using the continuous glucose monitoring system. *Diabetes Technol Therap* 7:233–240, 2005

Jovanovic L: Glucose and insulin requirements during labor and delivery: the case for normoglycemia in pregnancies complicated by diabetes. *Endocr Prac* 10 (Suppl. 2):40–45, 2004

Kaufman FR, Westfall E: *Insulin Pumps and Continuous Glucose Monitoring: A User's Guide to Effective Diabetes Management.* Alexandria, VA: American Diabetes Association, 2012

Kerr D, Macdonald IA, Heller SR, Tattersall RB: Alcohol causes hypoglycaemic unawareness in healthy volunteers and patients with type I (insulin-dependent) diabetes. *Diabetologia* 33:216–221, 1990

King AB, Armstrong DU: A prospective evaluation of insulin dosing recommendations in patients with type 1 diabetes at near normal glucose control: bolus dosing. *Journal of Diabetes Science and Technology* 1:42–46, 2007

King BR, Gross PW, Patterson MA, Crock PA, Anderson DG: Changes in altitude cause unintended insulin delivery from insulin pumps: mechanisms and implications. *Diabetes Care* 34:1932–1933, 2011a

King BR, Gross PW, Patterson MA, Crock PA, Anderson DG: Hitting the dartboard from 40,000 feet: a better chance with your eyes open! *Diabetes Technol Therap* 13:1075–1076, 2011b

Kirkman MS, Briscoe VJ, Clark N, Florez H, Haas LB, Halter JB, Huang ES, Korytkowski MT, Munshi MN, Odegard PS, Pratley RE, Swift CS: Consensus report: diabetes in older adults. *Diabetes Care* epub October 25, 2012:1–15. Accessed 10 February 2013. http://care.diabetesjournals.org/site/includefiles/dc12-1801.full.pdf

Kitzmiller JL, Buchanan TA, Kjos S, Combs CA, Ratner RE: Pre-conception care of diabetes, congenital malformations, and spontaneous abortions (Technical Review) *Diabetes Care* 19:514–541, 1996

Kitzmiller JL, Block JM, Brown FM, Catalano PM, Conway Dl, Coustan DR, Gunderson EP, Herman WH, Hoffman LD, Inturrisi M, Jovanovic LB, Kjos SI, Knopp RH, Montoro MN, Ogata ES, Paramsothy P, Reader DM, Rosenn BM, Thomas AM, Kirkman MS: Consensus statement: Managing preexisting diabetes for pregnancy. Summary of evidence and consensus recommendations for care. *Diabetes Care* 31:1060–1079, 2008

Klupa T, Benbenek-Dlupa T, Malecki M, Szalecki M, Steradzki J: Clinical usefulness of a bolus calculator in maintaining normoglycaemia in active professional patients with type 1 diabetes treated with continuous subcutaneous insulin infusion. *J Int Med Res* 3:1112–1116, 2008

Koivisto VA, Tulokas S, Toivonen M, Haapa E, Pelkonen R: Alcohol with meal has no adverse effects on postprandial glucose homeostasis in patients with diabetes. *Diabetes Care* 16:1612–1614, 1993

Kraus RM, Burkman RT Jr.: The metabolic impact of oral contraceptives. *Am J Obstet Gynecol* 167:1177–1184, 1992

Lange J, Arends J, Willms B: Alcohol induced hypoglycemia in type 1 diabetes. *Med Klin* 86:551–554, 1991

Maahs DM, Horton LA, Chase HP: The use of insulin pumps in youth with type 1 diabetes. *Diabetes Technol Ther* 12 (Suppl. 1): S59–S65, 2010

MacDonald MJ: Post-exercise late-onset hypoglycemia in insulin-dependent diabetic patients. *Diabetes Care* 10:584–588, 1987

Mannucci E, Ricca V, Mezzani B, Di BM, Piani F, Vannini R, Cabras PL, Rotella CM: Eating attitudes and behavior in IDDM patients: a case controlled study. *Diabetes Care* 18:1503–1504, 1995

Medtronic Diabetes: *Tape Tips and Site Management.* Northridge, CA: Medtronic Inc./Diabetes, 2011

Medtronic Diabetes: www.medtronicdiabetes.com/lifestyle/travel; www.medtronicdiabetes.com/lifestyle/equipmentinterference Accessed 10 February 2013

Mitchell T, Abraham G, Schiffrin A, Leiter L, Marliss E: Hyperglycemia after intense exercise in IDDM subjects during continuous subcutaneous insulin infusion. *Diabetes Care* 11:311–317, 1988

Nanchahal K, Ashton WD, Wood DA: Alcohol consumption, metabolic cardiovascular risk factors and hypertension in women. *Int J Epidemiol* 29:57–64, 2000

National Restaurant Association: *2012 Restaurant Industry Forecast.* Washington DC; National Restaurant Association, 2012

Nimri R, Wintrob N, Benazquen H, Ofan R, Fayman G, Phillip M: Insulin pump therapy in youth with type 1 diabetes: a retrospective paired study. *Pediatrics* 86:148–153, 1997

Northam EA, Anderson PJ, Werther GA, Warne GL, Adler RG, Andrewes D: Neuropsychological complications of IDDM in children 2 years after disease onset. *Diabetes Care* 21:379–384. 1998

Novo Nordisk A/S: *Levemir® (insulin detemir [rDNA origin]) injection Prescribing Information.* Novo Nordisk A/S, DK-2880 Bagsvaerd, Denmark, 2005–2012

Novo Nordisk A/S: *NovoLog® (insulin aspart [rDNA origin]) injection Prescribing Information.* Novo Nordisk A/S, DK-2880 Bagsvaerd, Denmark, 2002–2011

Okada M, Nomura S, Ikoma Y, Yamamoto E, Ito T, Mitsui T, Tamakoshi K, Mizutani S: Effects of postmenopausal hormone replacement therapy on A1C levels. *Diabetes Care* 26:1088–1092, 2003

OmniPod: www.myomnipod.com Accessed 10 February 2013

Pankowska E, Blazik M: Bolus calculator with nutrition database software, a new concept of prandial insulin programming for pump users. *J Diabetes Sci Technol* 4:571–576, 2010

Pankowska E, Blazik M, Groele L: Does the fat-protein meal increase postprandial glucose levels in type 1 diabetes patients on insulin pumps: the conclusion of a randomized study. *Diabetes Technol Ther* 14:16–22, 2012

Phillip M, Battelino T, Rodriguez H, Danne T, Kaufman F; European Society for Paediatric Endocrinology; Lawson Wilkins Pediatric Endocrine Society; International Society for Pediatric and Adolescent Diabetes; American Diabetes Association; European Association for the Study of Diabetes: Use of insulin pump therapy in the pediatric age-group: consensus statement from the European Society for Paediatric Endocrinology, the Lawson Wilkins Pediatric Endocrine Society, and the International Society for Pediatric and Adolescent Diabetes, endorsed by the American Diabetes Association and the European Association for the Study of Diabetes. *Diabetes Care* 30:1653–1662, 2007

Plotnick LP, Clark LM, Brancati FL, Erlinger T: Safety and effectiveness of insulin pump therapy in children and adolescents with type 1 diabetes. *Diabetes Care* 26:1142–1146, 2003

Price T, Rothman D, Taylor R, Avison M, Shulman G, Shulman R: Human muscle glycogen resynthesis after exercise: insulin-dependent and independent phases. *Journal of Applied Physiology* 76:104–111, 1994

Rabasa-Lhoret R, Bourque J, Ducros F, Chiasson J: Guidelines for premeal insulin dose reduction for postprandial exercise of different intensities and durations in type 1 diabetic subjects treated with a basal-bolus insulin regimen. *Diabetes Care* 24:625–630, 2001

Rabasa-Lhoret R, Garon J, Langelier H, Poisoon D, Chiasson JL: Effects of meal carbohydrate content on insulin requirements in type 1 diabetic patients treated intensively with the basal-bolus (ultralenter-regular) insulin regimen. *Diabetes Care* 22:667–673, 1999

Ratner RE, Dickey R, Fineman M, Maggs DG, Shen L, Strobel SA, Weyer C, Kolterman OG: Amylin replacement with pramlintide as an adjunct to insulin therapy improves long-term glycemic and weight control in type 1 diabetes mellitus: a 1-year, randomized controlled trial. *Diabet Med* 21:1204–1212, 2004

Richardson T, Weiss M, Thomas P, Kerr D: Day after the night before: influence of evening alcohol on risk of hypoglycemia in patients with type 1 diabetes. *Diabetes Care* 28:1801–1802, 2005

Rodin GM, Craven JL, Littlefield C: Eating disorders and intentional under-treatment in adolescent females with diabetes. *Psychosomatics* 32:171–176, 1991

Rosenn B, Siddiqi TA, Miodovnik M: Normalization of blood glucose in insulin-dependent diabetic pregnancies and the risks of hypoglycemia: a therapeutic dilemma. *Obstet Gynecol Surv* 50:56–61, 1995

Rovet J, Alvarez M: Attentional functioning in children and adolescents with IDDM. *Diabetes Care* http://www.ncbi.nlm.nih.gov/pubmed?term=Attentional%20functioning%20in%20children%20and%20adolescents%20with%20IDDM 20:803–810. 1997

Rutledge KS, Chase HP, Klingensmith GJ, Walravens PA, Slover RH, Garg SK: Effectiveness of postprandial Humalog in toddlers with diabetes. *Pediatrics* 100:968–972, 1997

sanofi-aventis: *Lantus (insulin glargine [rDNA origin] injection) solution for injection Prescribing Information*. Bridgewater NJ: sanofi-aventis U.S., 2007

sanofi-aventis: *Apidra (insulin gluslisine [rDNA origin] injection) solution for injection Prescribing Information*. Bridgewater NJ: sanofi-aventis U.S., 2009

Shashaj B, Busetto E, Suli N: Benefits of a bolus calculator in pre- and postprandial glycaemic control and meal flexibility of paediatric patients using continuous subcutaneous insulin infusion (CSII). *Diabet Med* 25:1036–1042, 2008

Sherman BM, Korenman SG: Hormonal characteristics of the human menstrual cycle throughout reproductive life. *J Clin Invest* 55:699–706, 1975

Simmons D, Thompson CF, Conroy C, Scott DJ: Use of insulin pumps in pregnancies complicated by type 2 diabetes and gestational diabetes in a multiethnic community. *Diabetes Care* 24:2078–2082, 2001

Sonnenberg G, Kemmer F, Berger M: Exercise in type 1 (insulin-dependent) diabetic patients treated with continuous subcutaneous insulin infusion: prevention of exercise induced hypoglycemia. *Diabetologia* 33:696–703, 1990

Strotmeyer ES, Steenkiste AR, Fooley TP Jr, Berga SL, Dorman, JS: Menstrual cycle differences between women with type 1 diabetes and women without diabetes. *Diabetes Care* 26:1016–1021, 2003

Swinburn BA, Sacks G, Hall KD, McPherson K, Finegood DT, Moodie ML, Gortmaker SL: The global obesity pandemic: shaped by global drivers and local environments. *Lancet* 378: 804–814, 2011

Tandem Diabetes: www.tandemdiabetes.com Accessed 10 February 2013

Thorell A, Hirshman M, Nygren J, Jorfeldt L, Wojtaszewski J, Dufresne S, Horton E, Ljungqvist O, Goodyear: Exercise and insulin cause GLUT-4 translocation in skeletal muscle. *Am J Physiol Endocrinol Metab* 277:E733–E741, 1999

Transportation Security Administration: *Travelers with Diabetes.* http://www.tsa.gov/traveler-information/passengers-diabetes Updated 28 January 2013. Accessed 10 February 2013

Turner BC, Jenkins E, Kerr D, Sherwin RS, Cavan DA: The effect of evening alcohol consumption on next-morning glucose control in type 1 diabetes. *Diabetes Care* 24:1888–1893, 2001

U.S. Department of Agriculture and U.S. Department of Health and Human Services: *Dietary Guidelines for Americans, 2010.* 7th ed. Washington, DC: U.S. Government Printing Office, 2010

Valensi P, Moura I, Le Magoarou M, Paries J, Perret G, Attali JR: Short-term effects of continuous subcutaneous insulin infusion treatment on insulin secretion in non-insulin-dependent overweight patients with poor glycaemic control despite maximal oral anti-diabetic treatment. *Diabetes Metab* 23:51–57, 1997

Walsh J, Roberts R: *Pumping Insulin: Everything You Need for Success on an Insulin Pump + a New Chapter on CGMs.* 5th ed. San Diego, CA: Torrey Pines Press, 2012

Wilson DM, Buckingham BA, Kunselman EL, Sullivan MM, Paguntalan HU, Gitelman SE: A two-center randomized controlled feasibility trial of insulin pump therapy in young children with diabetes. *Diabetes Care* 28:15–19, 2005

Wolpert H, ed: *Smart Pumping.* Alexandria VA: American Diabetes Association, 2002

Wolpert HA, Atakov-Castillo A, Smith SA, Steil GM: Dietary fat acutely increses glucose concentrations and insulin requirements in patients with type 1 diabetes: implications for carbohydrate-based bolus dose calculation and intensive diabetes management. *Diabetes Care* 35: 2012 Nov 27 [Epub ahead of print]

## CHAPTER 8

# Forms and Resources

All pump manufacturers provide pump education/preparation checklists; pump order forms, troubleshooting guides, and follow-up log forms. After the patient is trained by the manufacturer's certified pump trainer, the trainer will be happy to provide the original or a photocopy of the patient's pump brand-specific training checklist for your patient record.

The following pump education preparation and follow-up forms, guidelines, and checklists are examples of what you may find helpful; pump manufacturers have similar or other ones to help you and your patient prepare for and communicate during pump therapy initiation. Many blood glucose meters have the capability to download patients' data directly via email or phone, and patients may be able to supplement glucose meter data with carbohydrate intake, bolus doses, exercise notes, etc. The sample forms that follow may be adapted to suit your needs.

## Healthcare Professional Guidelines, Checklists, and Forms

These forms are completed by the HCP. File these forms in the patient's record.

## Insulin Pump Therapy Evaluation

- ■ Use to assess or evaluate and record a patient's readiness/preparation for pump therapy.
- ■ Can also be used to evaluate and record a <u>current</u> pump patient's needs for review and additional education.
- ■ Healthcare Professional (Physician and/or CDE) completes during pump therapy education process several weeks prior to date of pump training/pump start (which is conducted by the pump manufacturer trainer) OR during a routine or specific appointment for a <u>current</u> pump patient who is struggling with control and may need additional review and education.

## Insulin Pump Therapy Physician Start Orders/Prescription

- ■ Use to record prepump insulin regimen changes and orders for pump start.
- ■ Physician completes and provides to CDE and/or Certified Pump Trainer at least 5 days before pump start.

## Insulin Pump Therapy Follow-Up

- ■ Use to assess new pump patient's basic pump therapy knowledge.
- ■ Physician/CDE completes and determines patient's ongoing education needs and goals for success with pump therapy.
- ■ Physician/CDE can use on day of pump start and/or at first follow-up visit after day of pump start.

## Insulin Pump Therapy Telephone Follow-Up (two forms)

- ■ Use to record telephone information from patient during pump initiation period.
- ■ Physician or CDE uses to record one or several days of patient's SMBG results, carbohydrate intake, and bolus doses during pump initiation.

# Patient Guidelines, Checklists, and Forms

These forms are for the HCP to provide to the patient/parent of child patient. Some are to be completed by the HCP, and others are for the patient/parent to complete or use as needed.

## Insulin Pump Therapy Preparation Guidelines

■ Use to provide insulin changes/regimen and overall guidelines before and during the day of the pump start.

■ Physician completes several days in advance of the patient's pump start date. Photocopy after completion and file in patient's record.

## Insulin Pump Therapy Start Guidelines

■ This form summarizes the patient's pump start regimen and instructions.

■ Physician completes and provides a few days before or on the day of the pump start. Photocopy after completion and file in patient's record.

## Insulin Pump Therapy Record

■ This is a log form to record several days of SMBG readings, carbohydrate intake, carbohydrate bolus doses, correction bolus doses, and any other pertinent information that may affect target goals.

■ You may want to make several photocopies to provide to patient.

■ Patient uses this form to telephone or fax information to the clinician.

## Insulin Pump Therapy Information for Medical Procedure/Hospitalization/Surgery
NICHOLAS B. ARGENTO, MD

■ This form provides insulin pump therapy information to medical personnel in preparation for or during a patient's medical procedure, outpatient surgical procedure, or inpatient hospitalization.

■ Patient provides this form in advance of a medical procedure (X-ray, CAT scan, etc.), outpatient surgery, or inpatient hospitalization.

## U-500 Regular Insulin Instructions/Information
NICHOLAS B. ARGENTO, MD

■ Provide this form to the patient who will be using U-500 Regular insulin in a U–100-based insulin pump.

■ Physician completes and provides to patient as needed.

# Healthcare Professional Forms
## Insulin Pump Therapy Evaluation
## Pump Therapy Diabetes Self-Management Education
## Knowledge (Skills) Assessment/Plan

**Name** _____

**Date** _____

**Clinician/CDE** _____

### Assessment

**Patient understands/demonstrates:**

_____ Components of pump therapy

_____ Benefits and challenges of pump therapy

_____ Rationale of self-management using pump therapy (basal/bolus regimen)

_____ Need for frequent self-monitoring blood glucose (SMBG)

_____ Target blood glucose levels (has fasting, preprandial, postprandial targets)

Targets (mg/dl): Fasting _____ Preprandial _____ __ hr Postprandial_____

_____ Carbohydrate counting; has insulin-to-carbohydrate ratio[s] (ICR);

ICR: _____ units for _____ grams carbohydrate at _____ (meal[s])

ICR: _____ units for _____ grams carbohydrate at _____ (meal[s])

_____ Ability to use ICR to calculate meal/snack bolus doses

_____ Correction/sensitivity factor (CF); has factor(s)

CF: 1 unit of insulin lowers blood glucose _____mg/dl when BG <240 mg/dl)

CF: 1 unit of insulin lowers blood glucose _____mg/dl when BG >240 mg/dl)

_____ Ability to use CF(s) to calculate correction boluses

_____ Hypoglycemia: causes; symptoms; prevention; treatment (Rule of 15; glucagon)

_____ Need for glucagon prescription and/or unexpired glucagon

_____ Family member/significant other trained in use of glucagon

Name/relationship of person trained: _____

_____ Exercise/physical activity management guidelines

_____ Hyperglycemia: causes, symptoms, prevention, treatment (insulin, ketone testing)

_____ Has unexpired ketone test strips

_____ Sick day management guidelines

_____ Willingness to comply with medical recommendations

_____ Psychosocial adjustment (realistic expectations)

_____ Ability to use resources, e.g., support group, internet

_____ Financial resources (insurance or self-pay) for pump/supplies

**Patient has been shown basic features/functions of:**

_____ Pump brand models (indicate number of different pumps shown)

Brands/models_____

_____ Infusion set types/brands/models _____

_____ Insertion _____ Disconnection/Removal \_\_\_\_\_ Performed self-insertion

Handouts Provides _____

**PLAN**

_____ Patient is ready to choose pump and initiate insulin pump therapy per physician prescription and guidelines

_____ (Optional) saline start desired

_____ Recommended by clinician/CDE

_____ Requested by patient/parent (to inform pump company personnel)

_____ Requested by physician

_____ Refer to RD/CDE for carb counting education/review

_____ Patient requires additional education/follow-up prior to choosing pump

_____

_____

_____ Other _____

Notes/Comments _____

_____

_____

# Insulin Pump Therapy Physician Start Orders/Prescription

**Patient** _____

**Date** _____

**Physician Name** _____

Pump start date _____ Brand/model _____

Saline start? No _____ Yes _____ If yes, provide prescription for saline to patient

Saline start date _____ continue to _____

Insulin for pump _____ Humalog _____ NovoLog _____ Apidra

_____ Regular U-500 _____ Other _____

Insulin regimen <u>day before</u> pump start

_____ Usual basal/bolus regimen: _____ units long-acting insulin _____

_____ units rapid-acting insulin _____

_____

_____ New basal/bolus regimen:  _____ units long-acting insulin _____

_____ units rapid-acting insulin _____

_____ Discontinue basal insulin (___ Lantus ___ Levemir _____ Other _____)

_____ hours before pump start

_____ Continue injections of rapid-acting insulin every _____ hours before pump start

_____

If on pump therapy and switching to another brand/model of pump

_____ Continue current basal rates and bolus regimen

Other (as indicated below)_____

_____

If using oral diabetes oral medications (for type 2 diabetes)

_____ Continue current diabetes medication regimen

_____ Change oral diabetes medication regimen to _____

_____

Insulin regimen <u>day of</u> pump start

_____ Pre-breakfast: take usual injection of rapid-acting insulin only <u>with NO</u> basal (long-acting) insulin

_____

Starting basal rate(s)

_____ units/h (24 h)

Rate 1: 12 a.m. to ___ a.m. _____ units/h

Rate 2: ___ a.m. to ___ .m. _____ units/h

Rate 3: ___ a.m. to ___ .m. _____ units/h

Rate 4: ___ a.m. to ___ .m. _____ units/h

Target glucose levels (mg/d)

Fasting/premeal _____ ____

Other:    Postmeal _____

Bedtime _____

Nocturnal _____ a.m. _____

Insulin-to-carbohydrate ratio:     Bolus 1 unit for ____ g carbohydrate

Correction factor:   Bolus 1 unit for every _____ mg/dl > target blood glucose level/

range ____mg/dl

Insulin on board/Duration of insulin action: _____hours

Infusion set change

Change site and set every _____ to _____ days

_____,

MD/DO (prescribing physician)

Phone _____ Email _____

# Insulin Pump Therapy Follow Up

**Name** _____

**Date** _____

**Clinician/CDE** _____

**Patient understands/demonstrates:**

_____ Use of basic pump features and has been introduced to advanced features

_____ Infusion site selection, preparation, and hygiene

_____ Infusion set insertion and removal    Set type(s) _____

_____ Issues of daily living, e.g., wearing the pump, showering/bathing

_____ Exercise management guidelines

_____ Hypoglycemia causes, symptoms, prevention, and treatment (Rule of 15)

_____ Has unexpired glucagon

_____ Family member/significant other trained in use of glucagon

         Name/relationship of person trained: _____

_____ Hyperglycemia causes, symptoms, prevention, and treatment

_____ How and when to use ketone test strips (has unexpired strips)

_____ Sick day management guidelines

_____ Diabetic ketoacidosis (causes, prevention/treatment)

_____ Supplies to carry

_____ Problem-solving and troubleshooting guidelines

_____ Backup plans for time off the pump (has conventional therapy regimen)

_____ Who to call for clinical/diabetes questions, management, or help (physician, CDE/ diabetes educator [RD, RN, RPh, psychologist, exercise physiologist, other])

_____ Who to call for pump button-pushing, programming, or technical questions or help (pump manufacturer help line or other personnel as directed by pump company,)

_____ Who to call for pump supplies (pump manufacturer customer service, insurance company, other)

_____ Pump therapy follow-up guidelines

_____ Who to contact for followup during pump initiation period _____

_____ What to record: SMBG results, carbohydrate intake, bolus doses, activity, etc.

_____ When to contact follow-up staff: how often, times _____

_____ How to contact follow-up staff (phone, fax, e-mail)

_____

_____ Next clinical/diabetes follow-up office appointment scheduled for _____ with _____

_____ Attach copy of Certified Pump Trainer Training Checklist to maintain in patient record form.

# Insulin Pump Therapy Follow-Up

Name: _____
Day/Date: _____

Insulin Pump: _____     Insulin: _____
Glucose meter: _____

Target Blood Glucose: ___ mg/dL
Correction Factor: ___ mg/dL
Duration of Insulin Action: ___ hours

Basal Pattern: _____     Basal total: ___ u/day

| Basal rate | units/hour |
|---|---|
| 12:00 Midnight | |
| | |
| | |
| | |

Insulin: Carbohydrate Ratio: 1 unit: ___ g carbohydrate AND/OR Custom Boluses

1 unit: ___ g carbohydrate for breakfast     <Name>: ___     1 unit: ___ g carb, ___ % immed, 50% over ___ h
1 unit: ___ g carbohydrate for lunch         <Name>: ___     1 unit: ___ g carb, ___ % immed, 50% over ___ h
1 unit: ___ g carbohydrate for dinner        <Name>: ___     1 unit: ___ g carb, ___ % immed, 50% over ___ h

| Time | 12A | 1A | 2A | 3A | 4A | 5A | 6A | 7A | 8A | 9A | 10A | 11A | 12P | 1P | 2P | 3P | 4P | 5P | 6P | 7P | 8P | 9P | 10P | 11P |
|---|---|---|---|---|---|---|---|---|---|---|---|---|---|---|---|---|---|---|---|---|---|---|---|---|
| Basal rate u/h | | | | | | | | | | | | | | | | | | | | | | | | |
| Glucose mg/dL | | | | | | | | | | | | | | | | | | | | | | | | |
| Carbohydrate grams | | | | | | | | | | | | | | | | | | | | | | | | |
| Food bolus (u) | | | | | | | | | | | | | | | | | | | | | | | | |
| Correction bolus (u) | | | | | | | | | | | | | | | | | | | | | | | | |
| Set change | | | | | | | | | | | | | | | | | | | | | | | | |
| Comment | | | | | | | | | | | | | | | | | | | | | | | | |

Comments/Assessment: _____

Plan: ___ continue current regimen

OR ___ change regimen to:

Insulin: Carbohydrate Ratio: 1 unit: ___ g carbohydrate AND/OR Custom Boluses

1 unit: ___ g carbohydrate for breakfast     Custom Bolus 1: 1 unit: ___ g carb, ___ % imm, ___ % over ___ h
1 unit: ___ g carbohydrate for lunch         Custom Bolus 2: 1 unit: ___ g carb, ___ % imm, ___ % over ___ h
1 unit: ___ g carbohydrate for dinner        Custom Bolus 3: 1 unit: ___ g carb, ___ % imm, ___ % over ___ h

| Basal rate | units/hour |
|---|---|
| 12:00 Midnight | . |
| | . |
| | . |
| | . |
| | . |

Clinician Name: _____

# Insulin Pump Therapy Telephone Call FollowUp

**Patient** _____ **Date** _____

_____ Called as requested _____ Called because _____

_____ Was called by me

_____ To return patient's call _____ Because patient did not call as requested

**Current pump therapy regimen**

Pump brand:

____ ACCU-CHEK ____ Animas ____ Asante ____ Insulet ____ Medtronic ____ Sooil

____ Tandem _____ Other _____

Model: _____

Insulin: ____ Humalog ____ NovoLog ____ Apidra ____ Regular U-500 ____ _____

Basal rates:

(1) 12 a.m. to ___ a.m.: ____ units/h

(2) ___ .m. to _____ .m.: ____ units/h

(3) ___ .m. to _____ .m.: ____ units/h

(4) ___ .m. to _____ .m.: ____ units/h

(5) ___ .m. to _____ .m.: ____ units/h


Insulin-to-carbohydrate ratio          Correction factor

_____ 1 unit:15 g                      Add 1 unit for _____ mg/dl > _____ mg/dl

_____ 1 unit:12 g                      Subtract 1 unit for blood glucose < _____ mg/dl

_____ 1 unit:10 g

_____ 1 unit:_____ gm


SMBG record using _____ meter

Date:

| Time | 12:00 AM | 3:00 AM | Other___ AM | Pre-bfst | After bfst___ | Pre-lunch | After lunch | Mid-afternoon | Pre-dinner | After dinner | Bedtime |
|---|---|---|---|---|---|---|---|---|---|---|---|
| Blood glucose | | | | | | | | | | | |
| Carb grams | | | | | | | | | | | |
| Bolus dose | | | | | | | | | | | |
| Correction dose | | | | | | | | | | | |
| Total bolus dose | | | | | | | | | | | |

Date:

| Time | 12:00 AM | 3:00 AM | Other___ AM | Pre-bfst | After bfst___ | Pre-lunch | After lunch | Mid-afternoon | Pre-dinner | After dinner | Bedtime |
|---|---|---|---|---|---|---|---|---|---|---|---|
| Blood glucose | | | | | | | | | | | |
| Carb grams | | | | | | | | | | | |
| Bolus dose | | | | | | | | | | | |
| Correction dose | | | | | | | | | | | |
| Total bolus dose | | | | | | | | | | | |

Date:

| Time | 12:00 AM | 3:00 AM | Other___ AM | Pre-bfst | After bfst___ | Pre-lunch | After lunch | Mid-afternoon | Pre-dinner | After dinner | Bedtime |
|---|---|---|---|---|---|---|---|---|---|---|---|
| Blood glucose | | | | | | | | | | | |
| Carb grams | | | | | | | | | | | |
| Bolus dose | | | | | | | | | | | |
| Correction dose | | | | | | | | | | | |
| Total bolus dose | | | | | | | | | | | |

Date:

| Time | 12:00 AM | 3:00 AM | Other___ AM | Pre-bfst | After bfst___ | Pre-lunch | After lunch | Mid-afternoon | Pre-dinner | After dinner | Bedtime |
|---|---|---|---|---|---|---|---|---|---|---|---|
| Blood glucose | | | | | | | | | | | |
| Carb grams | | | | | | | | | | | |
| Bolus dose | | | | | | | | | | | |
| Correction dose | | | | | | | | | | | |
| Total bolus dose | | | | | | | | | | | |

Date:

| Time | 12:00 AM | 3:00 AM | Other___ AM | Pre-bfst | After bfst___ | Pre-lunch | After lunch | Mid-afternoon | Pre-dinner | After dinner | Bedtime |
|---|---|---|---|---|---|---|---|---|---|---|---|
| Blood glucose | | | | | | | | | | | |
| Carb grams | | | | | | | | | | | |
| Bolus dose | | | | | | | | | | | |
| Correction dose | | | | | | | | | | | |
| Total bolus dose | | | | | | | | | | | |

# Assessment

**Plan**

\_\_\_\_ Continue current regimen

\_\_\_\_ Change regimen to:

12 a.m. to \_\_\_\_ .m.: \_\_\_ units/h

\_\_\_\_ .m. to \_\_\_\_ .m.: \_\_\_ units/h

\_\_\_\_ .m. to \_\_\_\_ .m.: \_\_\_ units/h

\_\_\_\_ .m. to \_\_\_\_ .m.: \_\_\_ units/h

\_\_\_\_ .m. to \_\_\_\_ .m.: \_\_\_ units/h

Insulin:carbohydrate ratio          Correction factor

\_\_\_\_ 1 unit:15 g                    Add 1 unit for \_\_\_\_\_ mg/dl > \_\_\_\_\_ mg/dl

\_\_\_\_ 1 unit:12 g                    Subtract 1 unit for blood glucose < \_\_\_\_\_ mg/dl

\_\_\_\_ 1 unit:10 g

\_\_\_\_ 1 unit:\_\_\_\_\_ g

\_\_\_ Change SMBG regimen to _____

\_\_\_ Patient to call (date) _____ with SMBG results

\_\_\_ Patient scheduled with _____ on (date) _____

_____, MD/CDE

# Patient Guidelines, Checklists, and Forms
## Insulin Pump Therapy Preparation Guidelines

Name _____ Pump start date _____

Congratulations on your decision to start insulin pump therapy!

Several days or a week before your pump start day:

_____ Check all the contents of your pump box and make sure you have everything as indicated on the shipping list. Call the pump manufacturer with any problems.

_____ Review the user's manual and watch the instructional DVD.

_____ Confirm pump start date, time, and location with your physician/diabetes educator AND the pump company's Certified Pump Trainer.

Certified Pump Trainer _____ Phone _____

Time _____ Location _____ Phone _____

**The day before your pump start day:**

Insulin regimen

_____ hours before your pump start, discontinue

_____ (basal insulin) _____ injection(s)

Take _____ units of _____ hours before pump start

The night before your pump start day, add a middle-of-the-night glucose check

at _____ a.m. and correct if > _____ mg/dl

**Pump start day:**

Insulin

_____ Continue injections of your rapid-acting insulin _____

_____ Use your correction factor to correct a high blood-glucose reading

_____ 1 unit lowers your blood glucose _____ mg/dl

Blood glucose monitoring

_____ Continue to monitor your glucose as usual

_____ Add additional blood glucose checks _____

Allow 3 hours for training (or as directed by your trainer)

_____ Check your glucose, inject your meal bolus insulin to cover your breakfast, and eat your usual breakfast

_____ Use your insulin-to-carbohydrate ratio of 1 unit for ____ g carbohydrate

_____ Correct a high blood glucose level, as needed, with your correction factor

_____ 1 unit lowers your blood glucose _____ mg/dl

_____ Wear comfortable, two-piece clothing for your pump start

**Bring:**

_____ insulin (new, full vial or pre-filled cartridge) as prescribed by your physician

Insulin pump with all supplies sent to you, including:

- Pump user's manual and any literature, warranty information, etc.
- Pump batteries
- Pump cartridges/reservoirs
- Skin prep products
- Infusion sets and dressings/tapes

Glucose meter, strips/sensors, lancets, and lancing device
Calculator
Pen and paper
Food (lunch or snack)
Your usual treatment for hypoglycemia
Any other items as directed by your pump trainer _____

_____

_____, **MD/CDE**

# Insulin Pump Therapy Start Guidelines

**Patient** _____ **Date** _____

Congratulations on your decision to start insulin pump therapy! We will be speaking or communicating ___daily or ___every ____ days during the next few weeks, so please remember this when planning your schedule.

The following guidelines will help you during this start-up period:

Target blood glucose (goal):

■_____ mg/dl and, if applicable: _____

Blood glucose monitoring:

■Please check your blood glucose and record your results at the following times: 3:00 a.m., fasting, before each meal or snack, 2 to 2-½ hours after each meal or snack, and bedtime (about eight times daily).

■Keep a record of the glucose results, amount of carbohydrate consumed, and your bolus doses. Use any log book or form of your choice. For communication purposes during your pump initiation, it may be easier to write down the information instead of trying to read it from your meter's memory (unless you download and print your information).

Insulin type:

■___ Humalog ___ NovoLog ___ Apidra ___ Regular U-500

Basal rate:

■_____ units/hour. You will start with one rate for 24 hours.

■This rate will be changed as needed. Review your pump user's manual and have it handy so you will know how to add or change basal rates when directed to do so.

Exercise:

■Refrain from moderate to intensive exercise during this time unless directed otherwise. _____

Diet:

■Follow your usual diet (unless directed otherwise), using carbohydrate counting.

● Use your insulin-to-carbohydrate ratio(s) of 1 unit insulin for _____ grams of carbohydrate or (if applicable): _____

■During your pump initiation period, unless directed otherwise, please omit:

● Alcohol
● Chinese, Italian, Mexican, and any other high (or unknown amount of) carbohy-drate and/or high-fat meals/foods/beverages
● High-fat foods, including pizza, doughnuts, pastries, snack "cakes," pie, cake, and chocolate candy
● Foods not usually consumed
● Foods with unknown or undetermined amounts of carbohydrate or fat

Bolus:

■ Cover the carbohydrate you consume using your insulin-to-carbohydrate ratio(s), as described above. Example: You plan to eat 45 g carbohydrate, and your ratio is 1 unit for every 15 g. You would need to take a meal bolus of 3.0 units to cover the carbohydrate.

■ Based on your blood glucose level at the time, you may need to make adjustments in your bolus doses using your correction factor. See below

Hyperglycemia:

Correction factor:

■ Do not use your correction factor pre-meals until _____

■ ____ Do not take a correction bolus between meals unless directed otherwise.

_____

■ ____ Use your correction factor. For every _____ mg/dl over your target glucose, add 1 unit to your meal or snack bolus. Your pump can do the math for you and can calculate your correction bolus. Example: Your premeal target glucose is 100 mg/dl, and your correction factor is 50 mg/dl. Your premeal reading is 156 mg/dl. Because you are 56 mg/dl over your target of 50 mg/dl and 56 ÷ 50 = 1.1, you will need to add 1.1 units to your meal bolus to help lower your 156 mg/dl glucose level to your target of 100 mg/dl.

■ Bolus for high glucose readings no less than ____ h from your last bolus unless directed otherwise.

Ketones:

■ Make sure you have unexpired ketone test strips at home.

■ ____ Check for ketones when you have two consecutive blood glucose readings >240 mg/dl.

Hypoglycemia:

Pre-meal hypoglycemia and using your correction factor:

■ ____ For a glucose reading <80 mg/dl, subtract ___ unit(s) from your meal or snack bolus. Your pump can calculate this for you.

Between-meal hypoglycemia:

■ Follow the Rule of 15: A quick-acting source of 15 g carbohydrate, such as three to four glucose tablets, ½ cup juice, 8 oz skim/low-fat milk, or 4 to 6 oz non-diet soda, will raise blood glucose about 50 mg/dl in about 15 min. Recheck your glucose level after 15 min, and if you are still low, repeat the 15 g carbohydrate treatment.

■ Try not to overtreat because overtreatment can create a vicious cycle of low blood glucose, too high blood glucose, bolus, etc. Example: Your blood glucose is 60 mg/dl. Drinking ½ cup juice will raise it to about 110 mg/dl in about 15 min.

Infusion sets:

■ Change your set and site every 2–3 days, or as we discussed (every _____ days).

Call, fax, or e-mail your blood glucose, carbohydrate intake, and insulin bolus information daily, including weekends, unless directed otherwise.

Good luck! Remember, the next few weeks may be challenging, but learning pump therapy becomes easier every day, and all your efforts and hard work will be well worth it!

_____, MD/CDE

Phone _____ Fax _____ E-mail _____

# Insulin Pump Therapy Record

**Name** _____ **Date** _____

**Current pump therapy regimen**

Target blood glucose _____ mg/dl

Basal rates:     12 a.m. to ____ a.m. ____ units/h

_____ .m. to _____ .m.: ____ units/h

_____ .m. to _____ .m.: ____ units/h

_____ .m. to _____ .m.: ____ units/h

_____ .m. to _____ .m.: ____ units/h

_____ .m. to _____ .m.: ____ units/h

Insulin-to-carbohydrate ratio(s)

_____ 1 unit: ____ g

_____ 1 unit: ____ g

_____ 1 unit: ____ g

Correction factor

        Add 1 unit for _____ mg/dl above _____ mg/dl (target)

        Subtract ____ unit(s) for blood glucose <80 mg/dl

        Duration of insulin action ____ hours

Notes _____

_____

| Date | | | | | | | | | | | |
|---|---|---|---|---|---|---|---|---|---|---|---|
| Time | 12:00 AM | 3:00 AM | Other____ AM | Pre-bfst | After bfst___ | Pre-lunch | After lunch | Mid-afternoon | Pre-dinner | After dinner | Bedtime |
| Blood glucose | | | | | | | | | | | |
| Carb grams | | | | | | | | | | | |
| Bolus dose | | | | | | | | | | | |
| Correction dose | | | | | | | | | | | |
| Total bolus dose | | | | | | | | | | | |

| Date | | | | | | | | | | | |
|---|---|---|---|---|---|---|---|---|---|---|---|
| Time | 12:00 AM | 3:00 AM | Other____ AM | Pre-bfst | After bfst___ | Pre-lunch | After lunch | Mid-afternoon | Pre-dinner | After dinner | Bedtime |
| Blood glucose | | | | | | | | | | | |
| Carb grams | | | | | | | | | | | |
| Bolus dose | | | | | | | | | | | |
| Correction dose | | | | | | | | | | | |
| Total bolus dose | | | | | | | | | | | |

| Date | | | | | | | | | | | |
|---|---|---|---|---|---|---|---|---|---|---|---|
| Time | 12:00 AM | 3:00 AM | Other____ AM | Pre-bfst | After bfst___ | Pre-lunch | After lunch | Mid-afternoon | Pre-dinner | After dinner | Bedtime |
| Blood glucose | | | | | | | | | | | |
| Carb grams | | | | | | | | | | | |
| Bolus dose | | | | | | | | | | | |
| Correction dose | | | | | | | | | | | |
| Total bolus dose | | | | | | | | | | | |

| Date | | | | | | | | | | | |
|---|---|---|---|---|---|---|---|---|---|---|---|
| Time | 12:00 AM | 3:00 AM | Other____ AM | Pre-bfst | After bfst___ | Pre-lunch | After lunch | Mid-afternoon | Pre-dinner | After dinner | Bedtime |
| Blood glucose | | | | | | | | | | | |
| Carb grams | | | | | | | | | | | |
| Bolus dose | | | | | | | | | | | |
| Correction dose | | | | | | | | | | | |
| Total bolus dose | | | | | | | | | | | |

| Date | | | | | | | | | | | |
|---|---|---|---|---|---|---|---|---|---|---|---|
| Time | 12:00 AM | 3:00 AM | Other____ AM | Pre-bfst | After bfst___ | Pre-lunch | After lunch | Mid-afternoon | Pre-dinner | After dinner | Bedtime |
| Blood glucose | | | | | | | | | | | |
| Carb grams | | | | | | | | | | | |
| Bolus dose | | | | | | | | | | | |
| Correction dose | | | | | | | | | | | |
| Total bolus dose | | | | | | | | | | | |

*(This medical procedure form/letter created by Nicholas B. Argento, MD)*

# Insulin Pump Therapy Information for Medical Procedures/Hospitalization/Surgery

**A LETTER FROM: Pump patient in the hospital**

**TO: Anesthesiology/Surgery/Hospitalist**

**Patient name**: _____ **DOB:** _____

Date: _____

**I have type I diabetes or insulin-requiring type 2 diabetes and use an insulin pump,** which infuses insulin subcutaneously at a continuous programmed rate (the basal rate), and in addition is used to give multiple pre-meal or correction (for hyperglycemia) boluses. **I need basal insulin whether or not I am eating, which generally amounts to about ½ of my total daily insulin dose. "Sliding scale" insulin is not an adequate replacement for basal insulin requirements and can result in the development of iatrogenic diabetic ketoacidosis if used as my only insulin therapy.**

**My usual <u>total</u> daily insulin dose is: _____units.**

During surgery or hospitalization, my pump should generally not be touched except by me, unless a staff member familiar with my pump is available. My doctor may have recommended that I decrease the infusion rate slightly to prevent the possibility of low blood glucose while not able to eat before surgery. If the pump is discontinued, then basal insulin from the pump must be replaced by either continuous IV insulin infusion or a SQ regimen that includes scheduled basal insulin (NPH, glargine or determir) that amounts to ½ of my usual daily needs. If I am eating, then pre-meal rapid- or short-acting insulin (aspart, lispro, glulisine, or regular insulin) will also be needed. Sliding scale or correction insulin can be given to correct high blood glucose levels, usually pre-meal and sometimes before bedtime, in addition to basal and meal insulin.

If I develop low blood glucose before the operation, I can be given oral glucose tablets as treatment if available, because glucose tablets leave no residual material in the stomach. I would still be "NPO." If unable to take oral nutrients during the hospitalization, then IV glucose or IV nutrition is needed. It is possible my basal insulin dose may need to be decreased when not eating, but it cannot be stopped completely for the reasons already noted.

Care should be taken during transfer not to dislodge the infusion site from my skin. Please verify where the infusion site is before operations or procedures. The pump can be clipped to a gown or placed on the operating room table. If the pump infusion set becomes dislodged and cannot be restarted within 2 hours, or the pump sounds an alarm and no one familiar with my pump is readily available, then the pump will need to be stopped by removing the infusion set, and I will need to be switched to another insulin form/delivery using the guidelines above. **My blood glucose should be checked every hour while in the operating room, as well as before the operation and after the operation.** If I develop a low blood glucose (below 80 mg/dl) during the operation or in the post-op period, the insulin pump should generally be left alone and IV glucose should be given to correct the low blood glucose, and the blood glucose should be rechecked after 30 minutes. If the hypoglycemia persists, then the pump may need to be removed and basal insulin replacement started.

In general, I should be allowed to stay on the pump during hospitalization if possible, as long as I am alert and not sedated, and I have access to replacement pump supplies, and know how to make changes in my pump settings, and am physically able to do so. I understand that I must provide pump supplies for my pump, that the hospital cannot supply these. If I am not safe to operate the pump while in the hospital due to sedation or confusion, or the blood glucose is uncontrolled while on the pump, or the doctor thinks it is not safe for me to be on the pump, then the pump should be stopped, but I would need some basal insulin started immediately, for the reasons already noted above, in addition to a sliding scale and any nutritional insulin. If my need for insulin increases substantially, typically seen when there is need for steroids or IV nutrition, or with severe illness, then it may be better to switch me from the pump to another insulin form, but following the guidelines already given would allow this to be done safely and effectively.

Keeping blood glucose levels in a reasonable range is quite challenging while in the hospital. Everything relevant to the need for insulin changes in a hospital setting: activity decreases, stress increases, diet often decreases but almost always changes, and medications that increase the blood glucose (glucocorticoids, total parenteral nutrition, IV glucose, glucose containing IV medications) are often needed. Blood glucose levels above 200 mg/dl increase the risk of infection and impair healing, but low blood glucose presents a danger as well.

Please let me know when you order medicines or IV fluids that are likely to affect my blood glucose and need for insulin, or if I need to fast for a test or procedure.

Please call my diabetes doctor if you have questions. My diabetes doctor is:

Name: _____ Phone: _____

If you are having trouble keeping my blood glucose in an acceptable range during my hospitalization, please consider an endocrine consultation with a diabetes specialist, if available.

**I understand that while I am under your care, I need to follow the instructions that I am given from my medical team. I look forward to working with my medical team to do what I can do to keep my blood glucose controlled while under your care, so I can recover as quickly as possible.**

Patient signature: _____

Date: _____

*(This U-500 form created by Nicholas B. Argento, MD)*
# Patient Instructions for Use of
# U-500 Human Regular Insulin

**Patient:** _____

**Date:** _____

### U-500 Human Regular Insulin
■ is a very concentrated form of Regular human insulin.
■ has 500 units per 1 ml, which means that it has 5 times as many units in the same volume as any other insulin that comes in a vial or pen device. All other insulin from a vial or pen available in the United States contains 100 units per 1 ml (cc) (U-100). 1 ml or 1 cc is the volume in a full 100-unit syringe.
■ is prescribed for a patient who requires very high doses of insulin, generally more than 150–200 units per day.
■ takes twice as long to take effect compared to insulin lispro, insulin aspart, or insulin glulisine and lasts for a much longer time.
■ starts working to lower your blood glucose in about 30 minutes, peaks at 7 to 8 hours, and can last for up to 12 to 24 hours.

**All insulin syringes in the United States are marked for use with U-100 insulin, and insulin pumps are designed for use with U-100 insulin.**

**When using U-500 Regular insulin in a U-100 syringe, each 1 unit in the syringe contains 5 units of U-500 insulin.**

**When using U-500 Regular insulin in an insulin pump, each 'pump unit' actually is 5 units of U-500 insulin.**

Prescriptions for U-500 insulin must be written for the actual number of units to be used, which will be different than what the syringe or pump will indicate.

For example, 100 units twice a day of U-500 insulin would be measured as 20 units in a U-100 syringe. Here's the calculation: 100 units (prescribed dose of insulin) divided by 5 (to correct for the fact it is 5 times as concentrated as U-100 insulin) equals 20 units. To measure 100 units of U-500 insulin in a U-100 syringe, you would draw the U-500 insulin up to the 20 unit mark on the U-100 syringe.

In an insulin pump, to bolus 100 units of U-500 before a meal, you would set the pump to give (deliver) 20 units. Remember, each 'pump unit' when using U-500 in a pump is actually 5 units of U-500 insulin.

**Please use the table to convert the actual number of units that you will give when using U-500 insulin in a U-100 syringe or insulin pump. Or, you can simply divide the actual number of units to be given by 5.**

| Prescribed U-500 dose | Draw up in U-100 syringe | | Take this many pump units |
|---|---|---|---|
| 20 units of U-500 = | 4 unit mark in syringe | or | 4 pump units |
| 25 units of U-500 = | 5 unit mark in syringe | or | 5 pump units |
| 30 units of U-500 = | 6 unit mark in syringe | or | 6 pump units |
| 35 units of U-500 = | 7 unit mark in syringe | or | 7 pump units |
| 40 units of U-500 = | 8 unit mark in syringe | or | 8 pump units |
| 45 units of U-500 = | 9 unit mark in syringe | or | 9 pump units |
| 50 units of U-500 = | 10 unit mark in syringe | or | 10 pump units |
| 55 units of U-500 = | 11 unit mark in syringe | or | 11 pump units |
| 60 units of U-500 = | 12 unit mark in syringe | or | 12 pump units |
| 65 units of U-500 = | 13 unit mark in syringe | or | 13 pump units |
| 70 units of U-500 = | 14 unit mark in syringe | or | 14 pump units |
| 75 units of U-500 = | 15 unit mark in syringe | or | 15 pump units |
| 80 units of U-500 = | 16 unit mark in syringe | or | 16 pump units |
| 85 units of U-500 = | 17 unit mark in syringe | or | 17 pump units |
| 90 units of U-500 = | 18 unit mark in syringe | or | 18 pump units |
| 100 units of U-500 = | 20 unit mark in syringe | or | 20 pump units |
| 110 units of U-500 = | 22 unit mark in syringe | or | 22 pump units |
| 120 units of U-500 = | 24 unit mark in syringe | or | 24 pump units |
| 130 units of U-500 = | 26 unit mark in syringe | or | 26 pump units |
| 140 units of U-500 = | 28 unit mark in syringe | or | 28 pump units |
| 150 units of U-500 = | 30 unit mark in syringe | or | 30 pump units |
| 175 units of U-500 = | 35 unit mark in syringe | or | 35 pump units |
| 200 units of U-500 = | 40 unit mark in syringe | or | 40 pump units |

**Your insulin dose of U-500 Regular with a U-100 insulin syringe or insulin pump:**

Before breakfast: _____ units U-500 = _____ units in syringe or pump

Before lunch:        _____ units U-500 = _____ units in syringe or pump

Before supper:     _____ units U-500 = _____ units in syringe or pump

Before bedtime:    _____ units U-500 = _____ units in syringe or pump

**Your correction dose:**

Mealtime: add 10 units U-500 for every _____ mg/dl above _____.

Bedtime:   add 10 units U-500 for every _____ mg/dl above _____.

Check the table above to convert U-500 units to a U-100 syringe.

**Insulin pump settings:**

_____ Insulin on board function OFF

_____ Insulin on board function ON, with settings as follows:

Duration of action: 6 hours—Warning: the insulin-on-board feature will tend to underestimate how much active insulin is present.

_____ Don't use this function before bed.

**Target blood glucose setting:**

_____ mg/dl

**Insulin-to-carb ratio settings:**

Breakfast: 1 pump unit for _____ grams of carbohydrate

Lunch:     1 pump unit for _____ grams of carbohydrate

Supper:    1 pump unit for _____ grams of carbohydrate

**Correction (sensitivity) factor setting:**

1 pump unit (which is 5 units) will lower your blood glucose _____ mg/dl

**Other instructions:**

Check your blood glucose at 2:00 AM each night for the first week you use U-500 regular insulin.

Call the office if you are getting readings lower than 100 mg/dl at 2:00 AM.

_____

_____

_____

_____

_____

_____, **MD/DO**

# Insulin Pump Therapy Resources
WITH SUSAN L. BARLOW, RD, CDE

This list is not intended to be all-inclusive. The insulin pump and diabetes resources below may be of interest to both the healthcare professional and patient with diabetes. New insulin pumps and pump companies are on the horizon, so it's best to seek out the latest technology by surfing the internet and communicating with local diabetes educators, and pump manufacturers' sales representatives and clinical support staff. Product exhibits in professional diabetes and endocrinology conferences are also good sources of pump technology and information.

## Pump Manufacturers

Pump manufacturers provide specific guidelines for pump therapy initiation as well as the use of their pump(s). All manufacturers distribute pump supplies and accessories. Some manufacturers provide distribution and service to Europe and Asia.

ACCU-CHEK (Roche Insulin
   Delivery Systems, Inc.)
11800 Exit S Parkway, Suite 120
Fishers, IN 46037
1-800-280-7801
www.accu-chekinsulinpumps.com

Animas Corporation
200 Lawrence Drive
West Chester, PA 19380-3428
1-877-YES-PUMP (1-877-937-7867)
610-918-9524
www.animascorp.com

Asante Solutions, Inc.
352 East Java Drive
Sunnyvale, CA 94089
408-716-5600
www.asantesolutions.com

Cellnovo
Ethos, Kings Road
Swansea, SA1 8AS
+44-(0)20 3058-1250
www.cellnovo.com

Insulet Corporation
9 Oak Park Drive
Bedford, MA 01730
781-457-5000
www.myomnipod.com

Medtronic Diabetes
18000 Devonshire Street
Northridge, CA 91325-1219
1-800-MINIMED
(1-800-646-4633)
818-362-5958
www.medtronicdiabetes.com

Sooil Development Company, Ltd.
196-1 Dogok-Dong Kangnam-Gu
Seoul, Korea 135-270
+82-2-3463-0041
www.sooil.com
Distributed in the U.S. by:
DANA Diabecare USA
2601 N. Hullen Street
Suite 100
Metairie, LA 70002
1-866-342-2322
1-866-747-6645
504-889-9656
www.danapumps.com

Tandem Diabetes Care, Inc.
11045 Raselle St., Suite 200
San Diego, CA 92121
1-877-801-6901
858-366-6900
www.tandemdiabetes.com

**Note:** As of March 2009, the Smiths Medical/Deltec Cozmo pump is no longer available new, but the company honored its 4 year warranty for 2009 purchasers up to March 2013. Contact: www.delteccozmo.com OR 1-800-826-9703

## Pump Accessories

**Check the internet for additional new sites**

Insulin Pump Fashions
http://www.insulinpumpfashions.com

My Pumptastic
http://mypumptastic.com/
217-827-2034

Pump Wear Inc.
P.O. Box 633
Latham, NY 12110
1-866-470-PUMP (7687)
http://www.pumpwearinc.com/

Unique Accessories, Inc.
1625 Larimer Street
Suite 1206
Denver, CO 80202
1-800-831-8929
303-607-1298
www.uniaccs.com

## Insulin Pump Books for Healthcare Professionals

Evert AB: "Integrating Nutrition Therapy into Insulin Pump Therapy" in Franz MJ, Evert AB, eds: *American Diabetes Association Guide to Nutrition Therapy for Diabetes*. Alexandria, VA: American Diabetes Association, 2012

Kaufman FR, ed: "Tools of Therapy: Insulin Treatment: Continuous Subcutaneous Insulin Infusion," p. 68–73 in *Medical Management of Type 1 Diabetes, 6th ed*. Alexandria, VA: American Diabetes Association, 2012

Sherr J, Tamborlane W, Bode B: "Insulin Pump Therapy" in American Diabetes Association: *Therapy for Diabetes Mellitus and Related Disorders, 5th ed*. Alexandria VA: American Diabetes Association, 2012

Warshaw HS, Bolderman KM: "Advanced Carbohydrate Counting and Continuous Subcutaneous Insulin Infusion", pg 69–83 in *Practical Carbohydrate Counting: A How-to-Teach Guide for Health Professionals*. Alexandria VA: American Diabetes Association, 2008

Wolfsdorf JI, ed: "Insulin Infusion Pump Therapy" in *Intensive Diabetes Management, 5th ed*. Alexandria, VA: American Diabetes Association, 2012

## Insulin Pump Books for People with Diabetes

Kaplan-Mayer G: *Insulin Pump Therapy Demystified: An Essential Guide for Pumping Insulin*. Westport, CT: Pub Group West, 2003

Kaufman FR, Westfall E: *Insulin Pumps and Continuous Glucose Monitoring: A User's Guide to Effective Diabetes Management*. Alexandria, VA: American Diabetes Association, 2012

Walsh J, Roberts R: *Pumping Insulin: Everything You Need for Success On an Insulin Pump + A New Chapter on CGMs*, 5th ed. San Diego, CA: Torrey Pines Press, 2012

## Insulin Pump Consumer Magazine Publications for People with Diabetes

American Diabetes Association, *2013 Resource Guide*. Alexandria, VA: American Diabetes Association. www.diabetes.org 1-800-806-7801

**The following publications occasionally include insulin pump articles/ information:**

*Diabetes Forecast*
American Diabetes Association,
Alexandria, VA: American
Diabetes Association
http://forecast.diabetes.org/?loc=homepage_altcover
1-800-806-7801

*Diabetes Health*
Fairfax, CA
www.DiabetesHealth.com
1-800-234-1218

Diabetes Self-Management
New York, NY
http://www.diabetesselfmanage-
ment.com/magazine/
1-800-234-0923

## Diabetes Organizations and Associations

For more information about diabetes, including diabetes education, blood glucose target goals, carbohydrate counting, research, support programs for people with diabetes and their families and friends, and insulin pumps, contact the following organizations:

American Diabetes Association
  (ADA)
1701 North Beauregard Street
Alexandria, VA 22311
1-800-DIABETES or
1-800-342-2383
www.diabetes.org

American Association of
  Diabetes Educators (AADE)
100 West Monroe Street
Suite 400
Chicago, IL 60603
1-800-TEAM-UP4
(1-800-832-6874)
www.diabeteseducator.org

Juvenile Diabetes Research
  Foundation International
  (JDRF)
120 Wall Street
New York, NY 10035
1-800-223-1138
www.jdf.org

Centers for Disease Control and
  Prevention (CDC)
National Center for Chronic
  Disease Prevention and Health
  Promotion
1600 Clifton Road
Atlanta, GA 30333
1-800-311-3435
www.cdc.gov/diabetes

Insulindependence, Inc. (IN)
249 S. Hwy 101, 8000
Solana Beach, CA 92075
1-888.912.3837
http://insulindependence.org/

National Diabetes Education
   Program (NDEP)
One Diabetes Way
Bethesda, MD 20814-9692
1-888-693-NDEP
(1-888-693-6337)
www.YourDiabetesInfo.org

National Diabetes Information
Clearinghouse
1 Information Way
Bethesda, MD 20892–3560
1–800–860–8747
http://diabetes.niddk.nih.gov

## Insulin Pump Websites

Insulin Pumpers
www.insulin-pumpers.org

The Princess and the Pump
http://www.theprincessandthepump.com

## Diabetes Websites

**(may contain information related to insulin pump therapy)**

Children with Diabetes
www.childrenwithdiabetes.com

Close Concerns
www.closeconcerns.com

Diabetes Health
www.diabeteshealth.com

Diabetes in Control
www.diabetesincontrol.com

# Diabetes-Related Websites, Blogs, and Communities

**(may contain information related to insulin pump therapy)**

There are many websites with diabetes information that may also contain insulin pump information. Use search engine terms to locate diabetes- and insulin pump–related websites, links, and blogs. Most of these are patient-oriented, but the healthcare professional may also find them interesting.

This list of search terms is not all-inclusive:

- children with diabetes
- closed loop and diabetes
- college life and diabetes
- continuous subcutaneous insulin infusion
- CSII
- diabetes and insulin pump
- diabetes and pump research
- diabetes clinical trials
- diabetes life
- diabetes pump
- diabetes stories
- insulin pump
- insulin pump accessories
- insulin pump research
- living with diabetes
- my glucose
- pumping insulin
- pump therapy
- sweet life

## CHAPTER 9

# Tips from Pump Experts and Case Studies/ Success Stories

## Tips for Healthcare Professionals from Healthcare Professionals

These are tips from pump-experienced healthcare professionals (HCPs) that new-to-pump-therapy HCPs may find helpful.

1. Make sure you have the infrastructure support you need to effectively start a patient on a pump and maintain/follow the patient. The initial start-up involves, at a minimum, every-other-day, if not daily, contact with the patient to make basal rate adjustments and dosing recommendations. If you don't have time or want some help from experienced HCPs who have done this, do your homework. You may have pump-experienced Certified Diabetes Educators (CDEs) available in a local diabetes center or you can use one of the CDEs employed or contracted by the patient's pump company who can take over the follow-up management of the patient the first few weeks.

2. Take advantage of pump therapy literature, forms, guidelines, workshops, training sessions, etc., offered by the various pump manufacturers. Some are product-specific, while others are general—most have been edited through the years and are "tried and true." The pump companies are eager

to provide assistance because not only do they truly want the new-to-pump-therapy HCP and new pump patient to succeed; truthfully, they also want your business. Many HCPs new to pump therapy find the pump company assistance very helpful. And pump company sales and clinical (CDE) personnel are often pump wearers themselves and can provide real insight into their products and the entire patient pump therapy education and training process.

3. It's fairly unusual if, after a few weeks, your patient has only one basal rate. If that's the case, something's not right. Using just one basal rate for 24 hours/day is a waste of pump therapy. The patient may as well go back to MDI therapy, as that's a lot less costly than a $6000± glorified insulin pen or syringe.

4. Make sure the patient's basal rates are correct. Ask the patient to perform basal check tests until you've determined the correct basal rates. This can take several weeks. If the basal rates aren't right, no matter how well you think you (or another HCP) has calculated the insulin-to-carb ratio(s) and correction factor(s), they won't work right if the basal rates aren't right. A correctly determined basal rate allows the blood glucose to vary no more than 30 mg/dl hour-to-hour and overnight throughout the 24 hours. Determining the correct basal rates is a process that takes time and is a bit of a nuisance for the patient, but is well worth the effort.

5. At the patient's first visit following their pump training conducted by the pump company's personnel (ideally about a month after the pump start date) ask the patient to show you how some of the features work—such as changing a basal rate, setting a temporary basal rate, and changing the pump's clock time. If the patient's training was appropriate, the patient should be able to demonstrate understanding of basic features. And when you direct the patient to change or add a basal rate, the patient should be able to implement the change easily or with assistance from the user's manual.

6. Encourage your new pump patient to make/keep their quarterly follow-up appointments. Many pump patients become rather cavalier and over-empowered in their diabetes management and feel that seeing their physician "is a waste of time, since I know what I'm doing and my numbers are good." Stress the importance of obtaining routine

A1C values and other pertinent labs to fully assess the patient's overall health and the effects of diabetes on their renal and cardiac systems.

7. For the ultimate learning experience, ask one (or more) of the pump manufacturers to get you "hooked up" to a pump for 24 hours and simulate "pump life" to learn what your new pump patient is going through. You'll come away with a greater appreciation of the apprehension and challenges the patient experiences. And 24 hours is the right amount of time, because you'll be able to empathize with those first-day challenges of pump therapy, including eating, sleeping, showering, and learning new technology that literally keeps you [the patient] alive.

8. Stay updated with the current pump models, infusion sets, and prices—a general overview of information is all you need, as you can always refer patients to the pump company websites and/or sales reps for additional detailed information.

9. Be open-minded about who makes a good pump candidate. A college professor–type person with diabetes may be far less appropriate than a person with diabetes and no more than an eighth-grade education. It's the level of <u>diabetes</u> knowledge and the ability to problem-solve and troubleshoot diabetes challenges that are more important than the number of years of formal education. Some of the most successful pump patients are diabetes-savvy kids and high school dropouts, while college-educated patients can fail miserably on pump therapy.

10. Reinforce to patients how important it is for them to have a "backup plan." Pumps fail or break and it would behoove the patient to always be prepared, especially when traveling out of town or out of the country. Make sure, from the very beginning, you give your patient instructions for returning to MDI therapy, along with any necessary prescriptions for insulin pens or vials and syringes. And, in addition to your patient medical records, make sure the patient writes down their basal rates somewhere. Teach them that the sum of their basal rates is equal to the amount of basal insulin they can inject (once or split equally into two doses) using one of the long-acting insulin analogs. Don't assume that patients know that. And patients don't realize how quickly they can become ketotic without long-acting basal insulin. Experienced HCPs all have their pump patient stories: the pump patient who went to Brazil without a vial of insulin and syringes or

insulin pens and called, saying, "My pump broke. I have no syringes or a pen, and I have no idea what to do. Can you help?"

11. Attend a local diabetes insulin pump support group, if one is available. Volunteer or accept an invitation to be a speaker about a diabetes topic of interest, not necessarily pump-related. You'll be surprised at how much you learn about the challenges and benefits experienced by pump patients.

# Pump Tips for Patients from Patients
WITH SUSAN L. BARLOW, RD, CDE

These are tips from experienced pumpers that any pump patient, new or experienced, may find helpful.

## General

1. Learn the proper terms and names that are specific to pump therapy, such as basal, bolus, prime, suspend, and brand-specific words. For example, refer to the infusion set tubing as just that, and not "the line."
2. Upon receiving your pump, review the user's manual and view the instructional DVD before the pump training session. Jot down specific questions and notes to ask the pump trainer.
3. Do not be afraid of your pump. You have total control over it; it will only do what you program it to do. Remember this, and you will develop more confidence the longer you wear it. Respect your pump, treat it with care, and learn how to make it do what you want it to do. There are lots of resources to help you.
4. Check your blood glucose four to six times/day. Pump therapy is NOT a ticket to no–blood glucose testing land! Even though the pump can make living with diabetes easier, you still need to check your blood glucose in order to program the pump to perform its job.
5. With your pump trainer or educator, practice causing a warning/alarm to sound and/or vibrate so you can recognize it when it occurs. Learn how to take action to silence the alarm and fix the problem before you have a problem.
6. A copy of your user's manual is available online; know how to access it easily, or store the link in your computer or cell phone for easy access.

You may want to print out pages that you feel are important to keep with you when you are unable to access the internet or are away from home. At the very least, store a copy in your computer or smartphone, and print or photo-copy sections that you might want to refer to, including the warning/alarm section, especially if you need to learn alarm codes.

7. Know who to call for each type of problem. For a medical concern, call your healthcare professional. For a pump problem, call the pump manufacturer. Their toll-free number is located on the back panel of the pump and/or the companion remote control, glucose meter, or CGM device. Always carry emergency pump supplies. This includes a rapid-acting insulin pen, pen needles, and a vial/syringes, and a vial of rapid-acting insulin.

8. Have a backup plan in place, stored in your cell phone, computer, etc.— written down or recorded somewhere for easy access. There will be times when your pump may malfunction and/or when you need to be detached from the pump for more than an hour. When this occurs, you need to know what to do. It's easy to forget your pre-pump regimen. Make sure you have both rapid- and long-acting insulin available via an insulin pen and pen needles and/or vials and syringes so you can return to multiple daily injections until the issue is resolved.

## Wearing Options

1. There are many options available for wearing the pump, including cases, clips, pump-specific accessories, such as belts with pump cases, and leg garments, as well as specially designed clothing for pumpers. Check with the pump manufacturer for catalogs and suggestions. The internet is another source for pump accessories. The pump can be placed in the pockets of everyday apparel.

2. For both men and women, suggestions for wearing the pump include threading the tubing under the shirt or blouse and placing the pump in the pocket of a shirt or inside pocket of a suit jacket or blazer, a boot, money belt, cell phone case, change purse, fanny bag, gun holster, a pocket sewn into clothing, on a backpack strap, clipped to a belt, belt loop, or waistband (front or back).

3. Women may find that wearing the pump (in an infant sock) in their bra, either under the arm in the bra side panel or inside the cup, may be comfortable. Control-top panties, figure-slimming undergarments, panties

with "money or cell phone" pockets, and pantyhose also "anchor" the pump in place. Under dresses, the pump can be worn vertically in the small of the back. It can also be worn on the inside of the thigh or garter under long dresses. Some dresses have layered fabric or "cowl" necklines that can "hide" the pump. For sports, women can place or tape the pump to the front center of a sports bra.

4. Wearing the pump with long tubing inside your ankle- or high(er) sock works well for both women and men. If applicable, you can use your pump's remote device or cross your legs to deliver a touch bolus through your clothing.

5. If wearing the pump under clothing, placing the pump inside an infant sock prevents moisture buildup and adds to comfort. Infant socks are available in a variety of colors; look for thin, cotton socks without a crew top to eliminate bulkiness.

6. When shopping for a bathing suit or undergarments, women can place the pump in an infant sock and attach it to their own undergarments using a safety pin. This may be less bulky than a pump clip. Or, plan ahead and use the longest tubing so the pump can be placed on the floor or the dressing room seat/chair, or even wrapped around the neck so that it doesn't interfere with trying on the undergarments or bathing suit.

7. When showering, follow the pump manufacturer's guidelines for disconnecting and sealing (if applicable) your infusion set. Most pumps are watertight or waterproof. Your pump may come with a special device for showering or bathing to maintain watertightness. You may decide to not disconnect (for example, in a public gym or exercise club because you don't want to risk having your pump out of sight). You can then place your pump inside a small, resealable plastic bag, attach string at the top corners to hang it up or wear around your neck, and cut the lower corners of the bag to allow water to drain out. Other options include placing the pump inside a suction-cup soap dish or shower caddy.

8. For sleeping, try placing the pump in a specific location in the bed, such as next to you at your hip, clipped to the sheet or blanket, or inside a pajama, nightshirt, leisure pants, or nightgown pocket. You might like wearing a legband or armband. If placed under the pillow, the motor noise can be enhanced and may be disturbing. Restless sleepers may prefer longer tubing.

# Batteries

1. Always carry a spare battery(ies), especially if the pump uses an uncommon battery(ies) and/or battery charger, if applicable.
2. When changing batteries, always remove and discard the dead batteries before opening up a package of new batteries. Placing new batteries next to the old batteries can cause confusion, and the new batteries could end up being discarded by mistake.
3. If you need to replace your pump battery(ies) and your pump uses a commonly-found battery, such as an AA or AAA or one used in your cell phone, you can remove the other device's battery(ies) to use in your pump until you can obtain or purchase the much-needed pump battery(ies).

# Cartridge/Reservoir

1. When opening a cartridge/reservoir package, maintain sterile handling procedures. Placing the contents of the package on a paper towel makes viewing the contents easier and prevents rolling of the cartridge/reservoir.
2. Avoid possible contamination and bacteria transfer when filling the cartridge/reservoir or attaching tubing by not breathing or sneezing on or touching the top of the insulin vial or cartridge/reservoir components.
3. When filling the pump cartridge/reservoir, tap the side forcefully to move any air bubbles. Push up on the plunger and make sure you see the air travel through the hub of the needle and out at the tip into the insulin in the vial. It may be necessary to draw in additional insulin and tap again to push the air bubble(s) out. As the insulin in the vial is used, gently slide the pump cartridge/reservoir needle down and out of the vial to keep the needle tip inside the insulin in the vial.
4. Calculate the amount of insulin required to fill the cartridge/reservoir and the tubing (if applicable), and remember that a vial of insulin contains 1,000 units. Unless you change your cartridge every 2 days, do NOT pre-fill cartridges and store in the refrigerator, as insulin may begin to degrade when exposed to plastic within 48 hours. As handy or convenient as this may sound, resist the temptation!
5. Heat and temperature extremes can make the insulin less potent, causing high blood glucose readings. Insulin degradation can occur from the use of a Jacuzzi, sauna, or electric blanket. Anticipate the use of any of these, and

fill the pump cartridge/reservoir accordingly, i.e., with only a few days' usage, not a full cartridge.

6. Always insert a new cartridge/reservoir with room-temperature insulin. This will prevent air bubbles from forming in the tubing.

7. Discard the cartridge/reservoir needle in a sharps container or other approved refuse container. An empty plastic bleach or detergent bottle can be used. Secure the lid with masking tape and dispose in regular, not recyclable, trash.

## Priming

1. After priming, check the tubing daily for air bubbles. If you notice air in the tubing several hours or days after priming, you can disconnect the infusion set from your site and prime or deliver a bolus in "mid-air" to prime out the air space. To remove air bubbles from a disconnect-style infusion set, disconnect the infusion set from the site (never the pump), prime or bolus the air bubbles out in midair, and then reconnect.

2. One inch of tubing contains between 0.3 and 0.5 units insulin (varies depending on the brand of infusion set). With the introduction of new infusion sets, this amount may be different, so confirm with the set manufacturer. If using a non-disconnect infusion set or if it's inconvenient to disconnect your infusion set from your site and a large area of air bubbles is present, the amount of air (noninsulin) can be calculated, and a compensatory bolus can be delivered.

## Infusion Sites and Sets

1. There are many different infusion sets. Many sets are compatible with different brands of pumps even though they are made by a specific pump manufacturer. Try different sets to see what you might prefer. Some sets have a built-in disposable pod-like insertion device so that a separate inserter device isn't necessary. You may occasionally want to use a different infusion set for a specific reason. For example, a woman who wants to wear a clingy knit dress but doesn't want to have a "bump" (the plastic base of the Teflon cannula infusion set) showing through her dress can opt for a nonbase metal/steel needle set instead of her usual disconnect set. Work with your pump educator or trainer, and ask your pump manufacturer to send you samples of the various sets.

2. When using the abdomen for your infusion site, select tubing length that is longer than the distance from your abdomen to the floor, so that if the pump is dropped or falls off the waistband/belt, the infusion set will not come out. Restless sleepers may prefer longer tubing. Longer tubing for a non-disconnect infusion set may also be preferred for showering because the pump can be placed in a soap dish or shelf during the shower.

3. If you find the insertion painful, try numbing the skin with ice, a cold can of soda, a cold spoon, or an anesthetic cream, such as Emla or Ela-Max. The cream must be applied about 30 minutes before insertion, so keep this in mind when planning your site change.

4. Change your infusion sets every 2–3 days or per your healthcare professional or manufacturer instructions to avoid blockages, infection, and site issues.

5. "When in doubt, take it out." Change your infusion set when you have unexplainable persistent high blood glucose values. Do not allow high blood glucose levels to "go on," especially after you've given a correction bolus. If your glucose is not responding after 2 or 3 readings, change your site/set to rule out the possibility of an occlusion or scar tissue impeding the delivery of insulin. Hyperglycemia can be an indication that there is an absorption issue at the site.

6. Always change your site during daytime hours, when you will be awake for at least 4 hours after the set change. Therefore, if you have a site problem or set kink, you will not sleep through the nondelivery of insulin.

7. The infusion set tubing does not necessarily need to be changed with each site change. You can purchase infusion sets with extra needles or bases without tubing to control costs. Always change both the set and tubing if you have a site infection. "If in doubt, change it out."

8. When inserting the infusion set needle or cannula set introducer needle, stand rather than sit to prevent your skin from "bunching up" as you apply the dressing. Parents may find it best to insert the infusion set in a child who is lying down. "Stretching" the skin will also help with adherence and prevent the skin from feeling "pinched" below the adhesive.

9. For sweating at the site, use an antiperspirant at the site, allowing it to dry before attaching the infusion set dressing or tape.

10. To prevent needles/catheters from coming out, use an adhesive, such as IV Prep or Skin Prep. Spray adhesives include Bard Protective Spray,

Skin Prep, or 3M No Sting Barrier Spray. For stronger adhesion, try Mastisol, Skin Bond, or NuHope Adhesive. Pump manufacturers can provide a more inclusive list of appropriate products.

11. To assist with set adhesion, an infusion set can be sandwiched between two layers of dressing: apply a dressing to the site first, insert the needle/catheter through the dressing, and then apply the second set dressing/tape to the site's first layer of dressing.

12. For extra adhesion in securing an infusion set base with disconnecting tubing, perform your set insertion using the self-adhesive tape or set dressing. Fold an extra dressing or tape (larger than your infusion set self-adhesive tape) in half and cut a half-moon shaped piece out of it. When opened flat, there'll be a perfectly round open circle/hole in the center. Apply the open-center dressing/tape to the base dressing and your skin, then connect the infusion set tubing and proceed with filling the cannula or needle. The extra security is especially helpful when clothes shopping or changing clothes in a hurry—the infusion set is less likely to be accidentally "pulled out."

13. To secure the tubing to the site, make a "safety loop" before applying the infusion site dressing. The set will be less likely to come out if pressure is exerted on the tubing.

14. A waterproof bandage, HY tape, or Hypafix dressings can help keep infusion sets in place during exposure to water. A knee-sized waterproof adhesive bandage can also be used to cover the infusion site.

15. If you have difficulty removing the infusion set adhesive after changing your site, try a commercial adhesive remover product, such as Uni-Solve.

16. If using a Teflon cannula infusion set, remember to fill the cannula immediately after applying the site dressing. Follow the manufacturer's instructions. If you do not fill the cannula, you will miss part of your hourly basal rate, leading to high blood glucose levels.

17. If your pump doesn't offer a site/set change reminder, keep track of your site changes, and follow your healthcare professional's guidelines. Change a Teflon cannula set every 2–3 days and a metal/steel needle set every 1–2 days. If your pump doesn't have a set change reminder feature to help you remember to do this, use a calendar (e.g. set an alarm in your cell phone or other device) specifically for this, and you will never have problems remembering when it is time to change.

Remember, leaving the set in too long can cause poor insulin absorption, redness or tenderness at the site, high blood glucose levels, and, ultimately, tissue scarring.

18. Never disconnect the tubing from the top of the pump (pump "end") where it connects to the cartridge/reservoir until it's time to change the tubing. By disconnecting the tubing from the pump, you'll lose the insulin in the "hub" end of the tubing and will not receive several units of your basal rate or bolus dose. Also, if you've disconnected the tubing from the pump cartridge end and then reconnect it, the hub will very slowly fill back up with insulin, causing large air gaps in the tubing to occur (see Priming for tips on how to remove air gaps in the tubing).

19. Do not disconnect from your pump for more than an hour at a time. Your blood glucose levels will begin to rise quickly, as you no longer have long-lasting basal insulin in you.

20. When changing sites, make sure you use a site that totally healed from previous use. Try to choose sites a good inch away from the most recent site.

21. You may want to keep your most recent infusion set attached to your body until you determine the new site and set are working. Checking your blood glucose 2 to 3 hours after a set change will give you that confirmation. This is especially important if you've performed a routine site/set change and you know your most recent site and set had been working fine, you're short on supplies, and you've just used your last "emergency" infusion set to make the routine change.

22. Pets sometimes chew through infusion set tubing or dislodge an infusion set without your knowledge (during sleep or "rough and tumble" play with the pet). Always check your tubing to make sure it's connected at both ends. An insulin leak smells like a wet bandage, so do a scent check as well.

## Pump Settings

1. When setting maximum delivery amounts, take into account the total of your daily basal rates PLUS your daily boluses (meal boluses AND high blood glucose correction boluses). Remember to add a buffer amount (example: 10 to 20 units) for any potential increases in insulin needs, such as temporary basal increases, illness, or priming for air bubbles.

2. If applicable, practice use of the audio or touch bolus feature. Try using this feature while wearing the pump hidden discreetly under clothing.

3. If the pump is able to display its screen or backlight in a choice of time limits, choose the longer time initially. This choice uses more battery power but provides a longer screen display during the learning process. As you become more comfortable with using the pump, you can revert to the standard display time.

4. Learn about all the features of the pump, such as a temporary basal setting, but remember to stick with using the basic features initially. The "bells and whistles" can be reviewed and implemented after you've become comfortable with the basic functions of the pump. This step can take several weeks or months. Pump therapy is a process. Contact the pump manufacturer for pump operational questions or a review session on "advanced" features that you didn't use initially but feel confident using now.

5. Keep records of glucose readings, carbohydrate intake, bolus doses, exercise, stress, and other factors that can affect diabetes control. Look for glucose trends and patterns. Most pumps can be programmed with more than one set of 24-h basal rates. It may be necessary to initiate different 24-h basal rates for gym/exercise, high stress, travel, weekend versus weekday, or premenstrual days.

6. Limit use of the "Suspend/Stop Delivery" feature, if you use it at all. How much insulin are you "saving," i.e., not wasting, by putting your pump in suspend while you take a shower or bath? Consider your hourly basal rate at the time—1.0, 0.8, 0.7 u/hour?—your pump will be alarming for the time it's in "suspend."

7. Don't use the pump's suspend or "stop delivery" feature to treat hypoglycemia. It takes too long for the blood glucose to rise to make any significant difference. Putting your pump in the suspend mode for 15 to 20 minutes during a mild-to-moderate hypoglycemic event will not make a real difference in your blood glucose (will a basal rate of 0.6 units/hour really affect/lower your glucose to any measurable difference in the next 15 minutes?). People often forget to resume delivery and the result is hyperglycemia after several hours of non-delivery, especially if you ignore or don't hear the suspend/stop delivery alert/alarm.

8. Treat hypoglycemia following the Rule of 15: 15 grams of a fast-acting carbohydrate every 15 minutes until you reach your target glucose level.

Until you determine how to adjust your basal rate(s) for exercise, consider using a lower temporary basal rate for a few hours after exercise to <u>prevent</u> hypoglycemia.

## Basal Rates

1. When making basal rate changes or obtaining new basal rates from your healthcare professional, remember that the pump clock always starts at midnight (12 a.m.). Example: You have a regimen of three basal rates: 3 a.m. to 8 a.m.: 1.0 units/h; 8 a.m. to 4 p.m.: 0.7 units/h; and 4 p.m. to 3 a.m.: 0.8 units/h. This is actually a regimen of four basal rates because the start time of your first rate is midnight (12 a.m.). So, your actual basal rate program for 24 h is as follows: 12 a.m. to 3 a.m.: 0.8 units/h; 3 a.m. to 8 a.m.: 1.0 units/h; 8 a.m. to 4 p.m.: 0.7 units/h; and 4 p.m. to 12 a.m.: 0.8 units/h. To prevent any confusion, remind your healthcare professional to write any basal rate changes in this way, with the first rate starting at midnight (12 a.m.).

2. When you have advanced to using different basal patterns for gym/exercise, high stress, travel, weekend versus weekday, premenstrual days, etc., if your pump/software doesn't allow you to "name" the basal patterns, consider the order of the pattern numbers. Place the basal patterns in order of how often you would use them so you don't have to repeatedly review them before deciding which pattern is the one you want. Or, place them in "alphabetical order" numerically; for example, Pattern 1 is your everyday pattern, Pattern 2—exercise, Pattern 3—travel, Pattern 4—weekend.

3. After setting your basal rates, always review the settings. Check start times and basal rate amounts. Verify your pump's total with your hand-calculated total: add up your basal rates for each hour of the day. Your total should match your pump's total.

4. When making a basal rate change, multiply the net change in rates by the number of hours it will be in effect to get an idea of how much insulin you are increasing or decreasing. Use your correction/sensitivity factor (example, 1 unit lowers your blood glucose 50 mg/dl) to gauge how much the blood glucose is likely to change. For example, your basal rate change is an increase of 1.0 unit over 5 hours. So, in about 5 hours, 1.0 unit will likely to lower your glucose about 50 mg/dl.

5. When you have unexplained highs or lows, perform a basal rate check. Record your blood glucose at least 4 hours after the last bolus, fast for several hours while avoiding other factors that affect blood glucose (stress, exercise, etc.). Check your blood glucose over the next several hours to determine the effectiveness of your basal rate(s). If your blood glucose changes by more than 30 mg/dl from the initial reading, you may need to make a change in your basal rate(s).

6. Lead with the basal rate. It takes 2 to 3 hours after a change in the basal rate for the blood glucose to be affected, so the basal rate change should occur 1 to 2 hours before you want the change to occur.

7. Keep a record or list of your basal rates somewhere you can access easily, such as your cell phone, computer, or wallet. If your pump fails, you'll be unable to access the data and you'll need to know your basal rates to return to multiple daily injections. Better yet, memorize your daily basal pattern.

## Bolus Doses

1. If you need a refresher in carbohydrate counting, make an appointment with a Registered Dietitian/Certified Diabetes Educator (RD, CDE). Try to find one who has experience in pump therapy. Do NOT guess your food/carbohydrate intake. The beauty of an insulin pump is to be able to provide precision insulin delivery to cover what you will consume.

2. Make sure you use the pump's settings for your insulin-to-carb ratio(s) and correction factor(s). Don't guess at what your boluses should be—let the pump be your brain and do the math calculations.

3. Bolus for EVERYTHING you eat—snacks count as well as meals! A healthy person secretes insulin for every morsel of food eaten; to mimic a pancreas, your pump should do the same and you should remember to cover whatever goes into your mouth.

4. To prevent forgotten bolus doses, use your pump "bolus reminder" alarm/alert, if your pump has this feature. If not, decide on a specific meal/snack bolus delivery time, such as 15 minutes before eating.

5. High postprandial (after-meal) blood glucose levels can be lowered by taking your premeal bolus 15 to 20 minutes before the meal. But don't do this if your blood glucose is low or if you are not in control of the timing of your meal, such as in a restaurant. When dining out or

attending a celebratory event, it may be best to wait until the food "is in front of you" before you deliver a bolus. Delays in meal delivery happen often.

6. Learn how to cancel a bolus during delivery before you need to do this. Practice so that you will know what to do. Also learn how to check your pump's memory to see how much of the interrupted bolus you actually received.

7. If your pump is equipped with an extended bolus feature, such as an "extended" or "square wave" and a combination or "dual wave" bolus, work with your healthcare professional or pump trainer to learn how to best use this feature. Pumps that do not have an extended or combination bolus feature accomplish the same thing by using a temporary basal increase because an extended bolus is delivered during a pump's basal rate delivery. "Spreading the entire bolus out" or delivering a portion of it immediately and the remainder over several hours of time may be helpful for gastroparesis, high-fat meals/snacks (such as pizza and some desserts), high-fiber foods, and during parties or holiday meals. It may take several months of trial-and-error practice to develop a regimen that is right for you. Keep good records.

## Exercise/Sports

1. When engaging in active sports, do not disconnect the pump for more than 1–2 h without taking any insulin. Get specific guidelines from your healthcare professional for each type of sport or activity. Internet websites that contain pumper tips for exercise may be another resource, but remember that what works for one person may not apply to others. Various levels of a sport require different basal rates. The basal rate change is affected by the duration and intensity of the sport, your current glucose reading, the desired target glucose level, the time and amount of your last bolus, and the time, amount, and type of your most recent meal/snack. It will take several months of trial-and-error practice to determine what works best for you.

2. Check with your pump manufacturer for suggestions on wearing your pump during physical activity. There are many options; obtain accessory catalogs and surf the internet for ideas.

## Supplies to Carry

1. Follow your pump manufacturer's guidelines for carrying supplies. At minimum, <u>every day</u>, carry at least one of each item you need to keep your pump working. It's better to be safe than sorry. Remember that it's very likely there won't be anyone around close-by who will have the extra supplies you might need. This includes a complete set of batteries, insulin cartridge/reservoir, skin prep pad, infusion set, dressing/tape, vial of rapid-acting insulin, and medical identification card with emergency names and phone numbers. Additional helpful items include small folding scissors to cut dressing/tape, two bandages (for additional dressing adhesion), alcohol pads to cleanse dirty skin or dropped items, and insulin pens and pen needles (or insulin syringes and vials) of both rapid- and long-acting insulin in case of pump failure or pump loss/theft. Know appropriate insulin storage procedures. Check insulin and battery expiration dates frequently, and replace your skin prep (and alcohol pads, if you use them) often, too, so you are not surprised to open one that has dried out. And, keep a written record of your basal rates <u>somewhere</u>—if your pump fails, you won't be able to obtain the rates. Keep a record in your wallet, smart phone, computer, etc., and have a back-up plan!

2. Backup pump items can be kept in a cosmetic or pencil bag, small craft box, or clear plastic resealable baggie. Office workers can keep an additional supply in their locker or desk. A vehicle console or glove compartment or trunk is another place to store necessary items. Use caution when storing insulin/insulin pens, and follow the manufacturer's instructions.

3. Pump therapy does not guarantee perfect blood glucose control, so remember to include treatment for hypoglycemia in your emergency supplies. Suggestions include glucose tablets, glucose gel, small juice cans or boxes, cake icing in tubes, small bags or boxes of raisins, and individually wrapped jelly candies (containing 12–15 g carbohydrate per piece). Keep storage temperatures in mind, as the interior of a car or airline checked bag can become too hot or too cold and render your treatment useless.

4. Never leave your home without supplies! Whether you're going to be gone 30 minutes or for a month, always carry at least one of everything diabetes, and pump-related, most notably, treatment for hypoglycemia and an infusion set. A fall while walking, tubing caught in clothing while using the bathroom, the pump falling off you and cracking or breaking, along with mechanical car problems, and plane, train, bus, and automobile

delays can create unplanned and unforeseen emergencies. Insulin syringes and spare vials of both rapid- and long-acting insulin and/or insulin pens and pen needles are essential for overnight trips as well. It's better to over-pack and be safe than to be caught unprepared and in danger and sorry. Remember, you no longer have long-acting insulin in you when the pump stops working or the insulin delivery from the pump stops. Without basal insulin, a person with type 1 diabetes is headed toward diabetic ketoacido-sis in a matter of a few hours vs. a few days on MDI therapy. Be prepared!

# Case Studies/Success Stories

## Rob: Successful Pump Therapy Initiation in an Active Business Professional

26-year-old Certified Public Accountant

*Age at onset:* type 1 diabetes at age 17

*Height:* 72" (6')

*Weight:* 176 lb

*SMBG:* three to four times per day: premeal and bedtime (HS)

*Ranges:* 40–400 mg/dl; erratic control, nonspecific daytime pattern; fasting blood glucose (FBG) tends to be lower, 80–180 mg/dl, than other blood glucose (BG) readings

*A1C:* 8.2%

*Physical activity:* Winter: Basketball for 2 hours 2 days/week after work; Spring: Runs 30 min. 3 days/week after work; Summer: Bikes 1 hour or swims 30 min. 3 days/week after work; Fall: Runs 45 min. 3 days/week after work.

*Other:* Frequent hypoglycemia after physical activity. Admits to overtreat-ment with excess cola soda. Posthypoglycemia treatment SMBG results are >350 mg/dl. Consumes about 2,800 calorie/day based on "what I was told to do years ago. I tried carb counting but it's hard eating out for lunch or on long days at work when we do carry-out or order-in. I can count, obviously, as an accountant, but I pretty much eat the same amount of food at breakfast every day and I'm not a snacker. My lunch and dinner carb amounts vary, and I do a lot of guesstimating." Enjoys Chinese and Mexican food. Likes to sleep late on weekends and takes morning insulin 3 h later than on weekdays. On weekends, FBG is always elevated. Has supportive girlfriend.

*Current insulin regimen*
*Insulin lispro (Humalog) sliding scale:*
>   <100 mg/dl: 2 units
>   100–150 mg/dl: 4 units
>   151–200 mg/dl: 6 units
>   201–250 mg/dl: 8 units
>   251–300 mg/dl: 10 units
>   301–350 mg/dl: 13 units
>   a.m. Pre-breakfast: sliding scale (s/s) insulin lispro (usual dose 6 units);
>       10 units insulin glargine (Lantus)
>   Pre-lunch: s/s insulin lispro (usual dose 8 units)
>   Pre-dinner: s/s insulin lispro (usual dose 8–10 units)
>   HS: 10 units insulin glargine (Lantus)
>   TDD: average 41 units/day

## Pump therapy introduction

Rob is frustrated with his current control and restricted mealtime regimen; he wants more mealtime flexibility and less hypoglycemia. He has a colleague who wears a pump and likes it. Rob has concerns about wearing a pump during physical activity and sports, especially swimming. He asks his physician about pump therapy.

## Pump therapy preparation

**Clinician.** Rob's physician met with Rob and his girlfriend and explained pump therapy, demonstrated various water-resistant pump models and infusion sets, and provided written literature and a resource list of local pump manufacturer sales reps' contact information and pump manufacturer websites. She encouraged Rob to surf the internet to further explore insulin pump therapy, viewing sites included on the pump resources list. Rob's clinician then assessed Rob's expectations and self-care abilities, reviewed and provided target blood glucose levels, and provided contact information for Rob to schedule carbohydrate-counting sessions with an RD, CDE. Rob was asked to schedule a follow-up appointment several weeks following his RD, CDE appointment after learning and practicing carbohydrate counting.

**RD, CDE.** The RD, CDE taught carbohydrate counting to Rob and his girlfriend, determined an insulin-to-carbohydrate ratio (ICR) of 1:12 using Rob's food diary, and determined Rob's correction factor (CF) using his glucose records and the 1800 Rule (43 mg/dl rounded to 50 mg/dl). The dietitian had downloaded Rob's glucose meter and identified his blood glucose patterns, noting his weekday lunch postprandial numbers were consistently high (250–300 mg/dl) and his weekend numbers often ran lower (<225 mg/dl) than his weekday values. He had a lot of "lows" after exercise, and Rob admitted he "treated till feeling better" instead of following the "Rule of 15" (15 grams of carb every 15 minutes). Rob stated he was frustrated with the "ups and downs."

***Patient.*** Rob reviewed the written pump information/brochures and surfed the internet. He took advantage of a few pump manufacturer websites and their interactive virtual pump operations tools and programmed and "used" several pumps virtually (online). Rob attended one local pump support group meeting, where he met a 30-year-old successful pump wearer and softball coach. He obtained additional information on pump choices via the internet; met with two pump company sales representatives; and chose a pump. Rob's girlfriend helped him with contacting Rob's insurance company to verify coverage. The sales rep for Rob's pump helped Rob complete and obtain the necessary paperwork, including a letter of medical necessity and prescription from Rob's physician, and Rob learned about his insurance coverage (80% of $6500) for the pump and 3 months' (80% of $425) pump supplies. Rob learned carbohydrate counting and practiced successfully for 10 days before pump initiation. He met with the dietitian CDE again to verify his carb-counting skills had improved, and he obtained additional information on ethnic foods and how to identify "hidden" carbohydrate. Rob was able to successfully calculate premeal insulin lispro doses for unpredictable and varying amounts of carbohydrate in take-out and order-in lunches at his accounting firm. Rob's SMBG results improved and most of Rob's postprandial values were <250 mg/dl; occasionally, rather than frequently, he experienced a few high (>325 mg/dl) postprandial and low (<70 mg/dl) post-exercise values.

*Pump therapy initiation*
- ICR is 1:12
- CF is 50 mg/dl
- Premeal target glucose is 100 mg/dl
- Duration of insulin action: 3 hours
- Do not use CF for 3:00 a.m. SMBG
- No after-work sports for 7–10 days (until determining/fine-tuning basal rates)

*Prepump plan.* Rob's physician determined that Rob's insulin regimen for 24 h before the pump start should consist of continuing the insulin lispro doses and omitting the bedtime insulin glargine the night before the pump start.

## Day 1

■ Insulin lispro
■ Basal rate: 0.7 units/h (24 h)

*Clinician.* Rob's physician calculated the starting basal rate of 0.7 units/h × 24 h (41 units pre-pump TDD × 40% = 16.4 units ÷ 24 h = 0.68, use 0.7 units/h). She reviewed SMBG results, ICR, and CF; and provided Rob's starting basal rate, ICR, CF, duration of insulin action (3 hours), and target blood glucose values to the pump trainer (using a written form provided by the pump manufacturer) for Rob's pump settings. She gave pump initiation guidelines, including the need to omit after-work sports for 7–10 days during the basal rate adjustment period.

*Patient.* Rob viewed the pump instructional DVD the evening before his pump initiation.

■ 7:00 a.m. FBG: 202 mg/dl
■ Took 6 units insulin lispro to cover breakfast using 1:12 ICR; omitted morning insulin glargine dose.
■ Completed a 3-h pump training with the pump manufacturer's pump trainer in Rob's physician's office. Rob's girlfriend observed the training session and took notes.
■ Pump therapy initiated at 12:00 p.m. with basal rate of 0.7 units/h of insulin lispro for 24 h.
■ 12:00 p.m. pre-lunch: 134 mg/dl; 53 g carbohydrate, 4.4-unit bolus (53 ÷ ICR of 12 = 4.4); 0.7-unit correction bolus (34 mg/dl above target BG of 100 mg/dl) 34 ÷ CF of 50 = 0.7; total pre-lunch bolus dose is 4.4 + 0.7 = 5.1 units
■ 5:45 p.m. pre-dinner: 122 mg/dl; 67 g carbohydrate, 5.6-unit bolus, 0.4-unit correction bolus
■ 10:00 p.m.: 143 mg/dl

### Pump therapy follow-up and management

Rob's physician used the services of a local diabetes center CDE experienced with pump therapy to "follow" Rob—i.e., make basal and bolus adjustments per the physician's written and signed guidelines. Rob called the CDE daily to report SMBG results, carbohydrate intake, and bolus doses. Rob was reluctant to perform a 3:00 a.m. SMBG check the first 3 days (disliked waking up in the middle of the night and disrupting his sleep), but did so because he realized it was the best way to determine his overnight insulin needs.

## Day 2

- 3:00 a.m.: 132 mg/dl
- 7:00 a.m. FBG: 192 mg/dl; 42 g carbohydrate, 3.5-unit meal bolus, 1.8-unit correction bolus, total bolus = 5.3 units
- 11:30 a.m. pre-lunch: 111 mg/dl; 86 g carbohydrate, 7.2-unit bolus
- 6:00 p.m. pre-dinner: 134 mg/dl; 55 g carbohydrate, 4-unit bolus; 0.7-unit correction bolus (underbolused 0.6 units for carb); total bolus = 4.7 units
- 10:30 p.m.: 144 mg/dl

## Day 3

Implemented second basal rate (would see results on Day 4—see below):
- 3:00 a.m.: 139 mg/dl
- 6:45 a.m. FBG: 213 mg/dl; 42 g carbohydrate, 3.5-unit bolus; 2.3-unit correction bolus; total bolus = 5.8 units
- 11:30 a.m. pre-lunch: 156 mg/dl; 60 g carbohydrate, 5.0-unit bolus; 1.1-unit correction bolus; total bolus = 6.1 units
- 5:45 p.m. pre-dinner: 128 mg/dl; 76 g carbohydrate, 6.3-unit bolus; 0.6-unit correction bolus; total bolus = 6.9 units
- 10:00 p.m.: 119 mg/dl
- Based on results 48 h after start-up, the CDE added a higher basal rate of 0.8 units/h from 3:00 a.m. to 8:00 a.m. to reduce dawn phenomenon blood glucose excursions and decrease fasting blood glucose.

### *New basal pattern:*
- 12:00 a.m. to 3:00 a.m.: 0.7 units/h
- 3:00 a.m. to 8:00 a.m.: 0.8 units/h
- 8:00 a.m. to 12:00 a.m.: 0.7 units/h

## Day 4

- 3:00 a.m.: 112 mg/dl
- 7:00 a.m. FBG: 154 mg/dl; 45 g carbohydrate, 3.8-unit bolus; 1-unit correction bolus; total bolus = 4.8 units

- 11:30 a.m. pre-lunch: 117 mg/dl; 75 g carbohydrate, 6.3 unit bolus
- 5:30 p.m. pre-dinner: 96 mg/dl; 65 g carbohydrate, 5.5-unit bolus
- 10:00 p.m.: 123 mg/dl
- On Day 4, the CDE increased the 3:00 a.m. basal rate to 0.9 units/h.

## Days 5 and 6

New basal rates/pattern:
- 12:00 a.m. to 3:00 a.m.: 0.7 units/h
- 3:00 a.m. to 8:00 a.m.: 0.9 units/h
- 8:00 a.m. to 12:00 a.m.: 0.7 units/h

An increase in the 3:00 a.m. to 8:00 a.m. basal rate to 0.9 units/h resulted in FBG readings ±30 mg/dl within the target level of 100 mg/dl. Rob increased the frequency of his SMBG checks and continued to speak with the CDE daily the next several days.

## Day 7

Rob met with the CDE for a review of his SMBG results and observation of his third infusion site change. Rob, his girlfriend, the CDE, and the physician were pleased with his SMBG results. Rob was now ready to resume his after-work sports.

## Day 10

Sport days basal rates:
- 12:00 a.m. to 3:00 a.m.: 0.7 units/h
- 3:00 a.m. to 8:00 a.m.: 0.9 units/h
- 8:00 a.m. to 6:00 p.m.: 0.7 units/h
- 6:00 p.m. to 9:00 p.m.: temporary 50% decrease to 0.35 units/h
- 9:00 p.m. to 12:00 a.m.: resume 0.7 units/h

Ten days after pump initiation, Rob resumed his after-work swim and was instructed by the CDE to implement a temporary 50% decrease in his basal rate from 6:00 to 9:00 p.m. SMBG results were within target, and Rob did not experience post-swim hypoglycemia.

## Long-term follow-up

- Quarterly appointments with physician
- Annual appointments with RD/CDE

■ Basal program
   12:00 a.m. to 3:00 a.m.: 0.7 units/h
   3:00 a.m. to 8:00 a.m.: 0.9 units/h
   8:00 a.m. to 12:00 a.m.: 0.7 units/h
■ Basal total: 17.8 units
■ Average TDD: 39 units

Rob became accustomed to wearing his pump during biking, basketball, and running sports, but disliked wearing it for swimming. He called the CDE 2 months after pump start-up, and was advised to try disconnecting the pump during the half-hour-long swim and also discontinue the temporary 50% basal decrease. This proved to be successful. Rob continued to achieve SMBG results within his target range, with less frequent hypoglycemia and hyperglycemia. He continued to sleep late on weekends, and his weekend FBG results were similar to weekday FBG readings, within target range.

Three months after pump start-up, Rob's A1C dropped from 8.2% to 7.1%.

## Courtney: Successful Pump Therapy Initiation in a Female College Student

20-year-old college student
*Age at onset:* type 1 diabetes at age 11
*Height:* 64.5 inches (5', 4 1/2")
*Weight:* 141 lb
*SMBG:* usually 5–7 times/day: FBG, pre-meal, 2-h postprandial, HS. No specific pattern; frequent hypoglycemia
*Ranges:* FBG >200 mg/dl; premeal 50–270 mg/dl; postmeal 150–320 mg/dl
*A1C:* 7.9%
*Physical activity:* Weekday: mild-to-moderate, no formal exercise but has three 15–20 minute walks between college buildings for classes 5 days/week; Weekends: Bike rides, 2 hours/1 day/week; works 2 weekdays and every Saturday afternoon in the campus library restocking books and doing office (sedentary) work.

*Other:* Has mild retinopathy. States, "I'm either running high or low. I hardly ever have a normal blood sugar level, and I try really hard to do what's right. But I'm so busy with classes and work and it's hard to remember to count food and take my shots on time."

Was given carb-counting instruction 9 years ago. Admits, "I don't really follow anything specific. I thought I knew how to eat, but I think I need help. I'm tired of getting low blood sugars almost every day, and I have to eat when I don't want to." Courtney's parents are aware of her desire for a pump but are concerned about Courtney's commitment to the pump initiation process and her ability to learn how to use it. Courtney has concerns about wearing the pump, but one of her friends has a brother who uses a pump and Courtney is impressed that he doesn't have to "watch the clock and worry about running out of insulin and taking another shot at a certain time." Courtney said she wants more freedom in her schedule, but doesn't like the idea of having tubing "coming out of me and wearing a mini-computer 24/7." She admits to being frustrated with "everything."

*Current insulin regimen*
>    a.m.: Pre-breakfast: 7–10 units insulin aspart (NovoLog)
>    Pre-lunch: 5–7 units insulin aspart
>    Pre-dinner: 6–8 units insulin aspart
>    HS: 20 units insulin determir (Levemir)
>    TDD: average 41 units/day

## Pump therapy introduction

Courtney attended a local American Diabetes Association conference and visited the exhibit area. She saw insulin pumps at the booths and spoke with several pump manufacturer sales representatives and pump patients. Courtney read the information, watched a few DVDs, and called her physician for an appointment. She had questions about wearing the pump discreetly under her clothing but liked the idea of not having to worry about taking multiple injections and of eating when she desired instead of at specific times.

## Pump therapy preparation

**Clinician.** Courtney's physician explained pump therapy in more detail. He suggested that Courtney meet with pump sales representatives and consider a saline trial because of her concern about "how to wear the pump." He referred Courtney to an RD, CDE to learn carbohydrate counting, and provided a pump prescription to the pump company for insurance coverage and a saline trial prescription to Courtney and her pump trainer. The RD, CDE instructed Courtney in carbohydrate counting. She determined an ICR of 1:10 using the

Rule of 500 and a CF of 40 mg/dl using the 1800 Rule. The RD, CDE advised Courtney she might need to do bolus checks after beginning pump therapy to determine whether the insulin-to-carbohydrate ratio needs to be changed. She also arranged a follow-up appointment.

*Patient.* Courtney met with pump sales representatives and chose a patch/pod-type (tubing-free) pump. She worked with the RD/CDE on two occasions, learned and practiced carbohydrate counting for 1 month, and calculated premeal insulin doses. Courtney realized she had not known which foods affected her blood glucose levels and had some improvements in glucose readings: her high readings were lower, but the pattern was still erratic. Courtney's parents wanted to meet with the pump sales representative; therefore, an additional appointment was arranged. The appointment for pump initiation was arranged after the insurance company approved the pump. Courtney opted for a saline trial with her insulin pump. The week preceding her pump start with insulin she watched the pump instructional DVD and was trained by the pump manufacturer's pump trainer on the basic functions of the pump (filling the pod, pod placement/infusion set insertion, entering carb amounts, delivering and canceling a bolus—about 1½ hours of time) using saline. Courtney used her pump with saline for 3 days and wore it discreetly on her upper hip the first day, then switched to another pod and wore it on her upper arm. She delivered premeal saline bolus doses using the pump's remote device while continuing her insulin aspart and insulin detemir injections. Courtney thought the saline trial helped prepare her for "the real thing." She was glad she was able to "do a dry run" and wear the pod in several different sites. Much to her surprise, no one noticed the "little bump on my hip or upper arm—it was 'not a big deal' and easier than I thought it would be."

*Pump trainer.* The pump trainer instructed Courtney in basic pump functions and pod placement/infusion site insertion using saline. She suggested Courtney try wearing the pump on her hip or upper arm discreetly under clothing.

*Pump therapy initiation*
- ICR is 1:10
- CF is 40 mg/dl
- Premeal target glucose is 120 mg/dl
- Duration of insulin action: 3 hours

*Prepump plan.* Courtney's physician determined an insulin regimen for the 24 h before the pump start. Courtney was instructed to continue her premeal insulin aspart (NovoLog) doses, discontinue the insulin detemir the night before the pump start day, and add a 3:00 a.m. dose of 3–5 units insulin aspart, depending on her blood glucose level at 3:00 a.m.

## Day 1

- Insulin aspart
- Basal rate: 0.8 units/h × 24 h
- Cover breakfast with injection of insulin aspart, 8 units for 80 grams carb and FBG of 127 mg/dl (no correction insulin dose necessary)

*Clinician.* Courtney's physician calculated the starting basal rate of 0.8 units/h × 24 h. He used Courtney's basal insulin (insulin detemir) dose of 20 units ÷ 24 hours = 0.83, rounded down to 0.8 units/hour. He also verified using an alternate initial basal rate method. He calculated 50% of her total daily dose of 41 units = 20.5 units ÷ 24 hour = 0.85 units/hour, rounded down to 0.8 units/hour. He reviewed Courtney's SMBG results, ICR, and CF; provided the initial starting basal rate, insulin information, duration of insulin action (3 hours), and target blood glucose level (120 mg/dl) to the pump trainer; and gave Courtney pump initiation guidelines, including his fax number for follow-up. Courtney was advised to not use her CF the first 2 days of pump therapy.

*Patient.* Courtney injected insulin aspart, 8 units for 80 grams carb and FBG of 131 mg/dl (no correction insulin dose given) to cover her breakfast.

*Pump Trainer.* Courtney completed a second pump training/review (about 1½ h) with the pump manufacturer trainer in the physician's office. Since Courtney had already worn the pump with saline, she was familiar with some of its basic features. The pump trainer instructed Courtney in all the pump functions, e.g., programming basal rates, delivering combination boluses, etc., and reviewed the previously provided basic information and pump/pod infusion site insertion. She also provided additional tips on wearing the pump discreetly in the upper hips, lower abdomen, and upper arm areas under clothing.

- 6:00 a.m. FBG: 131 mg/dl
- Covered breakfast using 1:10 insulin-to-carbohydrate ratio (8 units for 80 grams carb)

- Pump therapy initiated at 11:00 a.m. with basal rate of 0.8 units/h
- 12:00 p.m. pre-lunch: 166 mg/dl; 45 g carbohydrate, 4.5-unit bolus; 1.15-unit correction bolus (vurrent BG = 166 mg/dl, 46 mg/dl above target of 120 mg/dl. CF = 40 mg/dl; 46 ÷ 40 = 1.15 units); total bolus = 5.65 units
- 6:00 p.m. pre-dinner: 88 mg/dl; 50 g carbohydrate, 5-unit bolus
- 10:00 p.m.: 216 mg/dl (no correction bolus—Courtney's physician wanted to see how the basal rate performed overnight to manage Courtney's blood glucose)

*Pump therapy follow-up and management plan*

Courtney faxed, called, or sent via her cell phone or computer her SMBG results, carbohydrate intake, and bolus information to her physician daily. He spoke or emailed with her each day and provided his recommendations.

## Day 2

- 3:00 a.m.: 222 mg/dl; no correction bolus
- 6:00 a.m. FBG: 229 mg/dl; 30 g carbohydrate, 3-unit bolus, no correction bolus
- 12:00 p.m. pre-lunch: 248 mg/dl
- Courtney emailed her results to the physician who advised her to use her CF to correct the 12:00 p.m. reading. Took 3.2-unit correction bolus to reach target of 120 mg/dl (248 mg/dl is 128 mg/dl above the target BG of 120 mg/dl; 128 mg/dl ÷ 40 [CF] = 3.2 unit correction bolus).
- 6:00 p.m. pre-dinner: 64 mg/dl; treated with 15 g carbohydrate; ate 60 g carbohydrate, 6-unit bolus
- 10:00 p.m.: 137 mg/dl

## Day 3

- 3:00 a.m.: 139 mg/dl
- 6:00 a.m. FBG: 124 mg/dl
- 11:00 a.m. pre-lunch: 156 mg/dl; 45 g carbohydrate, 4.5-unit bolus
- Courtney sent her results to her physician who told her to continue her current regimen. Her physician began to consider a midday basal check test to determine whether the basal rate is too high or whether Courtney is using too large a bolus to cover her noon meal.

■ 6:00 p.m. pre-dinner: 55 mg/dl; treated with 30 g carbohydrate; consumed 54 g carbohydrate, 5.4-unit bolus
■ 10:00 p.m.: 119 mg/dl

## Day 4

■ 3:00 a.m.: 112 mg/dl
■ 6:00 a.m. FBG: 120 mg/dl; 45 g carbohydrate, 4.5-unit bolus
■ 11:00 a.m. pre-lunch: 136 mg/dl
■ Courtney emailed her results to her physician who recommended that she perform a basal rate check to determine whether the 11:00 a.m. to 6:00 p.m. basal rate should be decreased. Courtney agreed to do the basal rate check, which required her to omit her lunch and perform SMBG every 2 h until 6:00 or 7:00 p.m.
■ 1:00 p.m.: 111 mg/dl
■ 3:00 p.m.: 82 mg/dl
■ 5:00 p.m.: 63 mg/dl. Courtney (over)treated with 35 g carbohydrate and ate an early dinner.
■ 8:00 p.m.: 145 mg/dl
■ 10:00 p.m.: 138 mg/dl

## Day 5

■ 3:00 a.m.: 141 mg/dl
■ 6:00 a.m.: 126 mg/dl; 45 g carbohydrate, 4.5-unit bolus
■ 11:00 a.m. pre-lunch: 140 mg/dl; 60 g carbohydrate, 6-unit bolus
■ Courtney sent her results to her physician who advised her to implement a lower basal rate of 0.7 units/h 11:00 a.m. to 6:00 p.m.

New basal rates:
■ 12:00 a.m. to 11:00 a.m.: 0.8 units/h
■ 11:00 a.m. to 6:00 p.m.: 0.7 units/h
■ 6:00 p.m. to 12:00 a.m.: 0.8 units/h

## Days 6–8

SMBG results within target range

## Long-term follow-up

Basal rates:
- ■ 12:00 a.m. to 11:00 a.m.: 0.8 units/h
- ■ 11:00 a.m. to 6:00 p.m.: 0.7 units/h
- ■ 6:00 p.m.–12:00 a.m.: 0.8 units/h
- ■ Basal total: 18.5 units
- ■ Average TDD: 36 units
- ■ Quarterly appointments with physician
- ■ Annual appointment with RD/CDE

Courtney enjoyed pump therapy and was thrilled with the consistency in her readings. She felt more energetic, and lost 3 lb, which she attributed to a decreased intake previously consumed for treatment of her recurrent prepump hypoglycemia. Four months after the pump initiation, Courtney's A1C dropped from 7.9% to 6.9%.

## Andrew: Successful Pump Initiation in a Late-Forties-Aged Engineer With Variable Work Hours

48-year-old product engineer who works three variable daytime shifts

*Age at onset:* type 1 diabetes at age 19

*Height:* 71 inches (5'11 1/2")

*Weight:* 201 lb

*SMBG:* seven to eight times per day: premeal, HS, and between meals during work hours; keeps detailed records, including pie charts and bar graphs

*Ranges:* FBG: 90–110 mg/dl; premeal: 130–180 mg/dl; HS: 110–160 mg/dl

*A1C:* 6.8%

*Physical activity:* Moderate physical activity; 1-h workout in gym using treadmill or running track 2 weekdays and 1 weekend day/week

*Other:* Treated recently for adhesive capsulitis at age 46. Is satisfied with his level of control but struggles to maintain target glucose levels. Has been counting carbohydrate for past 2 years. Is tired of multiple daily pen injections and finds it difficult to adhere to insulin regimen because of variable-shift work. Wants insulin pump for flexibility in lifestyle.

*Current insulin regimen*
> Pre-meal: insulin glulisine (Apidra) three times per day: pre-breakfast, pre-lunch, and pre-dinner
> Insulin-to-carbohydrate ratio: 1:5
> Usual doses range: 10–15 units/meal
> HS: 28 units insulin glargine (Lantus)
> TDD: average 64 units/day

## Pump therapy introduction

Andrew knows several people using insulin pumps. His physician has also recommended pump therapy. Andrew learned about the various pump models by speaking with pump users, researching the pumps on the internet, and comparing features in pump manufacturer literature and DVDs. He met with four manufacturer's sales representatives and chose a pump. Andrew arranged to meet with his physician to discuss pump therapy initiation.

## Pump therapy preparation

**Clinician.** Andrew's physician provided the necessary letter of medical necessity and prescription for insurance coverage.

**Patient.** Because he was already counting carbohydrate successfully, Andrew and his physician decided it was not necessary to meet with a dietitian. Upon receiving his pump, Andrew reviewed the user's manual and watched the instructional DVD. The pump manufacturer's pump trainer coordinated training in the physician's office.

*Pump therapy initiation*
- ICR is 1:5
- CF is 30 mg/dl
- Premeal target glucose is 100 mg/dl
- Duration of insulin action: 3 hours

**Prepump plan.** Andrew's current MDI regimen simulated pump therapy. Because the HS dose of insulin glargine acts as basal insulin, the bedtime insulin glargine dose was reduced by 50% the evening before his pump initiation. Andrew injected 14 units insulin glargine at 10:30 p.m. and was instructed to carefully monitor his glucose levels during the night.

## Day 1

- Basal rate: 0.6 units/h of insulin glulisine until bedtime; increase to 1.2 units/h at bedtime (11:00 p.m.)
- Omit exercise at gym for 1 week.

*Clinician.* Because Andrew's usual insulin glargine dose maintained his glucose levels within target, his physician calculated a starting basal rate of 1.2 units/h (of insulin glulisine) using the glargine dose as the basal rate (28 unit ÷ 24 h = 1.16, round to 1.2 units/h). Knowing that some of the preceding evening glargine dose may still be working during the first day of pump therapy, the physician initiated only 50% of the 1.2 units/h starting basal rate. Andrew's initial basal rate was calculated as 0.6 units/h, to be increased to 1.2 units/h at his bedtime, which was 11:00 p.m. The clinician instructed Andrew to call him each evening with his blood glucose and bolus dosages. He was told to continue using his CF of 30 mg/dl because it had proved successful with Andrew's prepump MDI regimen.

### Patient

- 3:00 a.m.: 125 mg/dl
- 6:30 a.m. FBG: 116 mg/dl (within target range)
- Andrew used his ICR of 1:5 to cover breakfast. Andrew was trained by the pump manufacturer's trainer and completed the 3-hour training by noon.
- 12:00 p.m.: 147 mg/dl; 45 g carbohydrate, 9-unit bolus; 1.6-unit correction bolus (47 mg/dl above target BG ÷ CF of 30 = 1.5); total bolus of 10.6 units (9.0 for carb + 1.6 correction)
- 6:00 p.m.: 156 mg/dl; 75 g carbohydrate, 15-unit bolus; 1.8-unit correction bolus; total bolus of 16.9 units
- Andrew called his physician, who advised him to continue his current regimen and reminded him to change his basal rate from 0.6 to 1.2 units/h at 11:00 p.m. Andrew did this.

### Pump therapy follow-up and management

## Day 2

- Basal rate: 1.2 units/h
- 3:00 a.m.: 111 mg/dl

- 6:00 a.m.: 74 mg/dl; 60 g carbohydrate, 11-unit bolus. Andrew's pump calculated a 12-unit bolus but the pump recommended reducing it to 11 units because his glucose was in a low-normal range.
- 11:00 a.m.: 98 mg/dl; 45-g carbohydrate snack, 9-unit bolus
- 3:00 p.m.: 72 mg/dl; Andrew felt mildly hypoglycemic and treated with 15 g carbohydrate
- 7:00 p.m. pre-dinner: 68 mg/dl. Andrew treated with 15 g carbohydrate; consumed 60 g carbohydrate for dinner, and used a 10-unit bolus to cover carbohydrate. His pump had calculated a 12-unit bolus but Andrew decided to reduce the bolus, thinking his basal rate might be too high. He called his physician, who agreed. Andrew was instructed to reduce his basal rate to 1.0 units/h × 24 h.
- 11:00 p.m.: 114 mg/dl

## Day 3

- Basal rate: 1.0 units/h × 24 h
- 3:00 a.m.: 101 mg/dl
- 7:00 a.m. FBG: 121 mg/dl. Andrew overslept and skipped breakfast.
- 9:00 a.m.: 92 mg/dl; 30 g carbohydrate, 4-unit bolus. Andrew realized he miscalculated his dose; he had given 2 units too little. He had ignored the amount his pump recommended because he was in a hurry and just "didn't want to verify if the pump calculation was right." He manually calculated his dose and didn't take advantage of his pump's calculations. He decided to wait until lunchtime to see whether his glucose would be higher than expected.
- 12:00 p.m.: 165 mg/dl; Andrew took a 2-unit correction bolus to correct the high reading; 62 g carbohydrate, 12.4-unit bolus
- 6:00 p.m.: 114 mg/dl; 56 g carbohydrate, 11.7-unit total bolus. Andrew called his physician, who was pleased with Andrew's results and advised him to continue his current regimen.
- 10:00 p.m.: 131 mg/dl; 1-unit correction bolus

## Day 4

- 3:00 a.m.: Andrew forgot to perform SMBG
- 6:30 a.m. FBG: 108 mg/dl; 46 g carbohydrate, 9.2-unit bolus
- 8:00 a.m.: 126 mg/dl

- 11:30 a.m.: 118 mg/dl; Andrew was too busy to eat lunch; omitted noon meal
- 3:00 p.m.: 95 mg/dl; 50 g carbohydrate, 10-unit bolus
- 8:00 p.m.: 64 mg/dl; Andrew had drunk two light beers during happy hour after work and munched on "a handful of pretzels." He did not take a bolus for the pretzels because he knew the alcohol might prevent his glucose from rising later if he were to become hypoglycemic. He treated with 15 g carbohydrate and called his physician. Andrew was advised to continue the current regimen and avoid alcohol the next few days during his pump initiation period.

## Day 5

- 3:00 a.m.: 144 mg/dl; 1.5-unit correction bolus
- 6:45 a.m.: 181 mg/dl; 2.7-unit correction bolus; omitted breakfast
- 8:30 a.m.: 262 mg/dl; Andrew called his physician, who asked him if he had changed his infusion site the preceding day. Andrew had not. He changed his infusion set and delivered a 5.4-unit correction bolus; consumed 45 g carbohydrate, 9-unit bolus.
- 12:00 p.m.: 116 mg/dl; Andrew was pleased with his reading and realized he must change his site every 2–3 days to prevent poor insulin absorption; 64 g carbohydrate, 13.3-unit bolus.
- 6:30 p.m.: 121 mg/dl; 66 g carbohydrate, 13.9-unit bolus
- 11:00 p.m.: 109 mg/dl

## Days 6–8

Andrew's glucose levels remained within target. He occasionally miscalculated his bolus doses and used his CF between lunch and dinner to decrease glucose elevations. He was able to skip some meals and eat at irregular times without adverse effects on his glucose readings. He was anxious to resume his exercise regimen and received his physician's permission to return to the gym.

## Day 9

- 1 h before exercise, at 5:00 a.m., Andrew implemented a 3-h, 30% temporary basal decrease for exercise
- 5:00 a.m.: 114 mg/dl; 30% temporary basal decrease. Basal rate 0.70 units/h × 3 h (30% reduction of 1.0 units/h = 0.7 units/h)

- 6:00 a.m. to 7:00 a.m.: 1 h exercise on running track and treadmill
- 8:00 a.m.: 89 mg/dl; resumed normal basal rate of 1.0 units/h; 45 g carbohydrate, 9-unit bolus
- 10:00 a.m.: 72 mg/dl; 15 g carbohydrate
- 12:00 p.m.: 101 mg/dl; 54 g carbohydrate, 10-unit bolus
- 6:00 p.m.: 131 mg/dl; 60 g carbohydrate, 10-unit bolus, 1-unit correction bolus
- 11:00 p.m.: 94 mg/dl

## Days 10–14

Andrew experimented with a lower temporary basal rate on his gym days (3 days/week). He reduced his 1.0 units/h basal rate by 40% to 0.6 units/h, and this reduction worked better than a 30% reduction. He had fewer episodes of hypoglycemia, and his glucose levels stayed within target range.

## Long-term follow-up

- Quarterly appointments with physician
- Gym days: 40% reduction in basal rate implemented 1 h before to 1 h after exercise (0.6 units/h × 3 h)
- Basal rate(s): 1.0 units/h
- Basal total: 24 units/day
- Average TDD: 54 units/day

Andrew was able to eat meals at times according to his work shift without having to worry about MDI injected insulin peak times. He was able to prevent post-exercise hypoglycemia using a temporary basal rate decrease. His 3-month post-pump start-up A1C level was 6.5%. Andrew felt he was able to maintain his excellent control with less effort (and less insulin) than when using MDI therapy.

## Tori: Successful Pump Initiation in a Mid-Thirties Beautician Using Split-Mixed Regimen

34-year-old beautician who works set part-time hours five days/week, three daytime shifts and two late-day evening shifts

*Age at onset:* type 1 diabetes at age 11

*Height:* 5'9"

*Weight:* 156 lb

*SMBG:* Five to seven times per day; premeal, HS, and between meals during work hours

*Ranges:* FBG: >165–200 mg/dl; premeal: 55–300 mg/dl; postmeal: 160–350 mg/dl; HS: 60–300 mg/dl. No specific pattern; complains of frequent hypoglycemia and hyperglycemia

*A1C:* 8.4%

*Physical activity:* Mild sporadic walking weekdays as beauty shop beautician and planned walks every other evening in neighborhood

*Other:* Nonproliferative retinopathy; past history of peripheral neuropathy (feet); admits to not following any specific meal pattern; has not been taught carbohydrate counting; has supportive husband with limited diabetes knowledge. Patient states: "I check my blood sugars a lot, and I'm either running high or low. I try to watch what I eat, and I exercise, but I still can't get things under control. I feel like I'm always 'chasing my insulin in the afternoons.' I get headaches from the lows, and I feel so tired when I'm high. I keep drinking cola or juice to bring up my blood sugars and I'm gaining weight from all those calories. Nothing I do seems to be working right. I had a customer who uses an insulin pump and she says she doesn't check her blood sugar as much as I do, and her A1C is lower than mine. I'd like to look into getting a pump. I think it would help me a lot. I just want to feel better. I'm exhausted, and I work just part-time five hours a day. I'm too young to be this tired."

*Current insulin regimen*
NPH bid: 16 units before breakfast (BB), 12 units bedtime (HS)
Regular insulin: sliding scale BB and before supper (BS):

       <100 mg/dl: 1 unit
       100–150 mg/dl: 2 units
       151–200 mg/dl: 3 units
       201–250 mg/dl: 4 units
       251–300 mg/dl: 6 units
       301–350 mg/dl: 8 units
       >350 mg/dl: 10 units

Usual two mealtime doses range: 2–8 units, 2 times/day
TDD: average: 36 units/day

## Pump therapy introduction
### Physician's Role

**Assessment:** Tori has erratic control; would benefit from pump therapy but physician wants to first try multiple daily injection (MDI) therapy to determine Tori's ability to troubleshoot and act on SMBG results. Tori is a bit reluctant to try a new insulin pen regimen but understands that the new regimen may help prepare her better for her ultimate goal of using an insulin pump.

**Plan:** Tori's physician (1) Introduced basal-bolus concept using MDI; explained pump therapy in more detail. (2) Implemented MDI therapy; established fasting, premeal, and HS blood glucose (BG) targets. (3) Referred Tori to RD, CDE to learn carb counting and be introduced to goals for successful pump therapy. (4) Referred Tori to Registered Nurse (RN), CDE for review/reinforcement of diabetes pump therapy information.

**Goal:** Improve Tori's A1C, self-monitoring blood glucose (SMBG) ranges/pattern, and her quality of life.

**Implementation of MDI therapy:**
MDI regimen using insulin glargine once/day and insulin aspart three times/day (tid): starting point based on split-mixed regimen
Insulin glargine: 30 u/day HS
Insulin aspart: three times/day (tid) pre-meal
      <100 mg/dl: 2 u
     100–150 mg/dl: 3 u
     151–200 mg/dl: 4 u
     201–250 mg/dl: 6 u
     251–300 mg/dl: 8 u
     301–350 mg/dl: 10 u
      >350 mg/dl: 13 u

**RD, CDE's Role:** Initial and 2nd visits over one month: Using food diaries and insulin doses, RD, CDE instructed Tori how to count carbohydrate and determined:
    ICR: 1 u: 12 g carb
    CF: 50 mg/dl

*Follow-up visit and phone/fax reviews:* Tori demonstrated understanding of carb counting; insulin-to-carb ratio and correction factor based on download of Tori's meter and her food diaries.

RD, CDE introduced pump therapy to Tori (two visits, first with Tori alone, second with Tori and her husband for review and glucagon training):

1. Explained pump therapy in detail, including the patient's responsibilities.
2. Showed Tori various pumps and infusion sets, and provided pump company literature, DVDs, and pump website links.
3. Suggested Tori call and meet with pump company representatives for additional information.
4. Suggested Tori attend local pump support group meeting to speak with current pump wearers. Provided date, time, and location of next pump support group meeting and encouraged Tori to attend.
5. Trained Tori's husband, with Tori observing, on use of glucagon. Instructed Tori to obtain prescription for glucagon from her physician.
6. Instructed Tori on the use of ketone test strips and importance of obtaining ketone test strips.

## Pump Therapy Preparation (over several months)

### RN, CDE:

1. Assessed, verbally and with written documentation, Tori's understanding and use of MDI regimen, carb counting, ICR, and CF.
2. Reviewed causes, symptoms, prevention, and treatment of hypoglycemia (Rule of 15 and the use of glucagon).
3. Reviewed causes, symptoms, prevention, and treatment of hyperglycemia, including the importance of ketone testing. Verified Tori had obtained ketone urine test strips as previously instructed.

**Patient:**
1. Tori demonstrated understanding of her MDI regimen, carb counting, and use of her insulin-to-carb ratio and correction factor.
2. Tori selected her pump model and informed her physician, CDE, and pump company representative.

3. With assistance from her physician and pump company representative, Tori completed her insurance paperwork (covered at 80% under her husband's insurance plan). Tori's physician completed Tori's pump prescription form.

**Physician:**

At three months, Tori's physician obtained an A1C value, as it had been three months since Tori was switched from a split-mixed regimen to MDI therapy. Her A1C had improved from 8.4% to 7.9%.

Tori's pump was delivered and signed for at her home. Tori called her physician and RD, CDE to schedule her pump start in conjunction with the pump company trainer. The pump company trainer had called Tori to schedule the training. Tori reviewed the pump user manual and start-up guide and became familiar with the button-pushing prior to her scheduled pump start.

## Pump Start:
## On the Day Preceding the Pump Start:

Tori's physician discontinued her HS glargine dose; substituted HS glargine with NPH insulin. HS dose: 10 units of NPH (about 1/3 of 30 units, Tori's total daily insulin glargine/basal insulin dose)

## Pump start day:

Based on her pre-pump glargine dose of 30 units/day, Tori's physician calculated Tori's starting basal rate: 30 u/day ÷ 24 hours = 1.25 units/hour starting basal rate. Tori's physician did not reduce the starting basal dose, as her A1C was still elevated.

ICR: 1 u: 12 g carb

CF: 50 mg/dl (not to be used first 2 days unless otherwise directed by the RD, CDE who would be following/managing Tori during her pump initiation.

Target blood glucose: 100 mg/dl (FBG, premeal)

Additional desired pump features (indicated on Pump Start Order Form): Duration of insulin action: 3 hours

Tori ate her usual breakfast using her ICR and CF.

She arrived at the training site (physician's office) at 8:30 a.m. for training by the company pump trainer. The pump training was completed in 3.5 hours at 12 noon. Tori was now wearing the pump and infusion set.

■ 12 noon: 166 mg/dl. ate 45 g carb lunch, 3.75 unit bolus.

■ 3:00 p.m.: 188 mg/dl; no food, no bolus

■ 6:00 p.m.: 129 mg/dl, 64 g carb, 5.3 unit bolus

■ 9:00 p.m.: 72 mg/dl; drank 20 g carb juice

## Day 2

Basal rate: 1.25 units/hour × 24 hours

■ 12:00 a.m.: 144 mg/dl

■ 3:00 a.m.: 158 mg/dl

■ 7:00 a.m. 202 mg/dl; 60 g carb breakfast, 5.0 unit bolus

■ 12:00 noon: 166 mg/dl; 45 g carb lunch, 3.75 unit bolus

■ 3:00 p.m.: 188 mg/dl

■ 6:00 p.m.: 129 mg/dl; 90 g carb dinner, 7.5 unit bolus

■ 9:00 p.m.: 72 mg/dl, drank 15 g juice.

■ Next day (**Day 3**) 12:00 a.m. 96 mg/dl

Tori had been instructed to not correct any BG elevations. Her RD, CDE and physician wanted to determine how her basal rate was working. Elevated BG between 3:00 a.m. and waking indicates Tori has dawn phenomenon and needs a higher basal during 3:00 a.m. and 7:00 a.m; will increase basal rate to 1.4 units/hour (about a 12% increase). Low BG in evening after dinner indicates she may need a lower basal rate OR a different insulin-to-carb ratio. Will ask Tori to skip dinner and perform a basal rate check test. She may need a lower basal rate from 6:00 p.m. to 12:00 a.m. (midnight).

## Day 5

■ 3:00 a.m.: 116 mg/dl; will begin higher basal rate of 1.4 units/hour for 4 hours, 3:00 am to 7:00 a.m.

■ 7:00 a.m.: Basal rate (resumed) 1.25 units/hour; 101 mg/dl; 44 g carb breakfast, 3.7-unit bolus

■ 12:00 noon: 133 mg/dl; 60 grams carb, 5.0 unit meal bolus; 0.6-unit correction bolus; total bolus = 5.6 units

■ 3:00 p.m.: 108 mg/dl

■ 6:00 p.m.: 117 mg/dl; performing basal rate check test, skipped dinner, checked blood glucose hourly.

- 7:00 p.m.: 99 mg/dl
- 8:00 p.m.: 86 mg/dl
- 9:00 p.m.: 72 mg/dl; drank 15 g carb (juice)
- Next day (**Day 6**) 12:00 a.m.: 101 mg/dl

Tori is thrilled with her daytime BG results. The basal rate check test indicates her basal rate of 1.25 units/hour between 6:00 p.m. and midnight is too high, as her blood glucose decreases hourly. She needs a lower basal rate during those hours. Tori's physician advises her to implement a rate of 1.0 units/hour (about a 20% decrease) between 6:00 p.m. and 12:00 a.m. (midnight).

## Day 9

- Basal rates: Midnight to 3:00 a.m.: 1.25 units/hour
- 3:00 a.m. to 7:00 a.m.: 1.4 units/hour
- 7:00 a.m. to 6:00 p.m.: 1.25 units/hour
- 6:00 p.m. to 12:00 a.m. (midnight): 1.0 units/hour
- 3:00 a.m.: 96 mg/dl
- 7:00 a.m.: 102 mg/dl; 60 grams carb, 5.0 unit bolus
- 12:00 p.m; 109 mg/dl; 60 grams carb, 5.0 unit bolus
- 6:00 p.m.: 122 m/dl: 75 grams carb, 6.25 unit bolus
- 9:00 p.m.: 135 mg/dl

## Next day (Day 10)

12:00 a.m.: 129 mg/dl.
Tori is very happy with her BG results and can't believe how her energy level has increased.

Overall, Tori began with one basal rate and after a week and a half, had three basal rates.

**Long-term follow-up:** At three months, Tori's A1C level had decreased from 7. 9% to 6.9%. She felt better, had more energy, and fewer headaches. She also lost 3 pounds and attributes that to less juice for the "lows" she was having mid-afternoon. Tori said pump therapy "was a bit of work even before I started it [referring to the switch over from a split-mixed regimen to MDI], but it was worth it.

## CHAPTER 10

# What Lies Ahead: Insulin Pumps of the Future

NICHOLAS B. ARGENTO, MD
KAREN M. BOLDERMAN, RD, LDN, CDE

Some of us have had the privilege, both as patients with type 1 diabetes and practicing healthcare professionals (endocrinologist, dietitian) with a strong interest in insulin pumps, to see many beneficial changes become available in diabetes therapy and technology. We have experienced dramatic advances in diabetes care and management, particularly those of us diagnosed in the 1960s. A diagnosis of type 1 diabetes had once been a death sentence. Insulin, the miracle drug that saves lives, would not have been available to anyone prior to 1922, and was not generally available until several years later (Bliss 1982).

Let's consider the diabetes landscape of 1965. At that time, disposable insulin syringes were not yet available. Those of us diagnosed then had to either boil glass syringes or store them in a jar of alcohol. Disposable needles had been introduced and could be attached to the glass syringe, which at least avoided the need to sharpen multiuse needles. It wasn't until a few years later that the totally disposable insulin syringe with attached needle became widely available. This somewhat eased the burden of injecting insulin. However, the insulin available (U-40, U-80) was of animal (bovine or porcine) source, which generated higher titers of antibodies and a higher incidence of local reactions than currently available insulins. Basal insulins (lente, NPH, PZI [protamine zinc iletin], ultra-lente) had significant peaks that could be variable and unpredictable, and mealtime insulin (regular, semi-lente) was of slower onset and longer duration than was desirable (Hirsch 2005). A more important limitation was that the only way to assess current glycemia was with urine glucose testing. Laboratory blood glucose tests could be used to check a single fasting or random blood glucose level only every few months. Self-monitoring of blood glucose and the A1C test were not yet available, so there really was no effective way for either the patient or the healthcare professional to know what the current blood glucose was or to assess the degree of overall glycemic control. Tight blood glucose control, which was not of proven benefit, was nearly impossible to achieve for the average patient. It amounted to driving on a twisting mountain road with eyes closed. Efforts to achieve better blood glucose control were often rewarded by frequent hypoglycemic reactions, requiring family, friends, teachers, coworkers, and romantic partners to become experts on the recognition and treatment of hypoglycemia.

The prognosis for avoiding complications for a person with type 1 diabetes in the 1960s was certainly not encouraging. And what if one did develop diabetes complications? Laser therapy for diabetic retinopathy was not yet available, so the risk for developing blindness was high (American Diabetes Association 2002). The important connection between hypertension and nephropathy was not yet fully appreciated, and treatment options for hypertension were somewhat limited, and did not include ACE (angiotension converting enzyme) inhibitors or ARBs (angiotensin receptor blockers). Renal dialysis had become available to treat renal failure (Blagg 2007) but transplant medicine was in its infancy (Morris 2004). There were not effective treatments generally available for painful diabetic neuropathy, coronary artery disease, or erectile dysfunction.

Some people living with diabetes had their first experience with a portable glucose meter in the 1970s. A wedge-shaped hand-held lancet was used to get a very large drop of blood from the finger, a lancet that left cuts that could take days to heal, and after three minutes the user was able to see a blood glucose reading. A home glucose meter was introduced in the early 1970s (Mendosa 2012), but few knew about it. For most, it wasn't until 1980–1981 when those who knew about it had access, could afford it, and were able to purchase their first glucose meter. One of the first home blood glucose meters available was a device that was about 6 inches long, required a very large drop of blood and the use of a small spray bottle of water to rinse off the blood after waiting one minute, then at two to three minutes, the result appeared. The device had a somewhat limited range, no memory, and cost about $400, quite a sum at that time, a sum that was often "out of pocket" since it was infrequently covered by insurance. Fortunately, the painful lancet wedge had been replaced by a spring-loaded automatic lancing device, referred to by some patients as "the guillotine." The lancets and glucose test strips were not inexpensive, either: a vial of 50 glucose test strips cost nearly $100. Despite these limitations, an indispensable tool in any effort to achieve euglycemia was becoming accessible and available: self-monitoring of blood glucose.

The insulin pump was first introduced as a backpack model in 1963, and by 1971, the pump was smaller (Mendosa 2012) but still large (weighing about a pound) compared with today's modern pumps. A limited number knew about and could access this new technology. In 1981, a young medical student with type 1 diabetes had read studies about a new device to deliver insulin, the continuous subcutaneous insulin infusion pump. He contacted an endocrinologist at Johns Hopkins Hospital in Baltimore, Maryland, and was told that he should plan on spending seven to eight days in the hospital at the start of pump therapy. The pump measured about 6 × 4 × 2 inches and weighed about eight ounces. It had only one basal rate, though it could be programmed to deliver extra units at a later time. One had to specify the duration of and delay in starting the infusion (in minutes) on a daily basis; for example, 2 units to infuse over 180 minutes, to start in 420 minutes. The pump required a rechargeable battery, with a very short battery life, so that one needed to have three batteries: one charging, one in the pump, and one ready to go. The infusion set was a straight needle that was manually inserted at an angle and taped down. Though primitive by modern standards, this and other early insulin pumps allowed better glucose control, with less hypoglycemia, and improved flexibility. Rapid strides in pump technology added dosing and safety features, a reduced size, and an improved ease of use and have made pump therapy available to a wider group of patients (Pickup 2012).

So what is different as of 2013? Unlike in 1965 or 1981, there is no longer any doubt that tight glycemic control can prevent or delay the development of diabetic complications (Diabetes Control and Complications Trial Research Group 1993). There are obvious technologic advances in pump therapy, many of which have been reviewed in this book—pumps are smaller, more discreet, and menu-driven with control buttons that are more intuitive. Multiple basal rates can be set, and fractions of units can be delivered in a variety of different patterns. Infusion catheters are far more comfortable and are either tubeless or easily detachable. Battery life is now measured in weeks, not hours. Continuous glucose monitoring is available, whether as a separate device or integrated with the pump. But more importantly, a pump has gone from essentially being a fancy way to deliver insulin, best used by 'high operating' patients, to being a 'smart pump'—a sophisticated diabetes management device that can help a patient figure out how much insulin to give, and give many options on how to give it. Healthcare professionals also benefit from pump software to review and evaluate what patients are actually doing, or sometimes not doing. Pump software can assist in recognizing patterns so that necessary changes can be made. An insulin pump is now a much more powerful and patient-friendly tool than when first introduced in the 1970s. Because pumps are more sophisticated, patients can be less tech-savvy.

Where are pumps going, and where do they need to go? The ultimate goal is to have a fully functional closed-loop insulin infusion pump, one that takes the patient out of the loop, with the capability to infuse glucagon as rescue therapy. Short of that, what would we, as pumpers and healthcare professionals dedicated to helping pump patients, like to see? An incomplete list of features, many of which are far along in development or are available in some places, would include:

- Tubeless or "patch pumps" that have a flatter profile and smaller footprint, with separation of the insulin reservoir from the pump mechanism from the infusion platform, thus allowing temporary removal of the reservoir, especially during ascent in flight (King 2011) or whenever it might be unsafe or inconvenient to wear it, like during sporting events or intimate relations.
- Consolidation of devices, with a cell phone device that can serve as a smart phone with downloaded carbohydrate applications, a glucose meter with pattern recognition software, a remote pump controller, and a continuous glucose monitor receiver. This is the unmet need that is requested most often, short of a closed-loop implanted device.
- A truly integrated insulin pump and continuous glucose monitor that can suspend delivery when hypoglycemia is detected and resume infusion once hypoglycemia is resolving, with a low rate of false hypoglycemia alarms
- Dual-chamber pumps, with the possibility of pairing insulin with glucagon or pramlintide.
- Bigger cartridge/reservoirs that can hold 400–500 units of insulin, to accommodate insulin-resistant patients.

- Adjustable insulin concentration, to be able to set the concentration of insulin as U-100, U-200, U-500, or any other concentrations that are likely to become commercially available, which would minimize potential for error and allow easier use of pumps in our highly insulin-resistant patients. For safety reasons, it might be possible to make such a feature accessible only by the HCP or pump manufacturer. The availability of higher insulin concentration(s) could also lead to the development of smaller pumps for those who are not insulin resistant.

- More concentrated rapid analogs, in U-200 or U-500 concentration vials or pre-filled cartridge/reservoirs, to allow quicker onset and thus, better mealtime coverage than is possible with U-500 regular in highly insulin-resistant pump patients.

- Louder alarm capability integrated into the pump. Many patients with hearing loss have difficulty hearing current pump alarms, which are usually high-pitched, and may not feel a vibration alarm, especially when asleep. It would seem technologically feasible to make a much louder alarm, such as used by an alarm clock, to be triggered when the patient does not respond to the usual alarm.

- Talking pumps, with basic functions accessible with voice prompts, for our visually impaired patients, as well as larger font potential when needed.

- For all pumps to be fully travel friendly, that is, fully immune to any interference from airport security screening or changes in altitude, and fully waterproof.

- More complex smart pump bolus settings. For example, fat content adjustments that are based either on estimated grams of fat, or a semi-quantitative high-fat setting. It would be important to allow immediate bolusing to cover some of the carbohydrates, and 1 or even 2 different delayed boluses, with a capability of starting a delayed bolus several hours in the future. Protein adjustments for high-fat meats would be helpful, which could be in ounces or grams or just >4 ounces, also giving a delayed bolus. Activity adjustment settings that would allow a reduction in the net bolus for moderate (30%) and vigorous (60%) activity would also be useful.

- A temporary percentage adjustment to all boluses, much as we can now do with a temporary basal rate. For example, if a patient was given a steroid injection into a large joint, it is likely that the blood glucose will be higher for 3–7 days afterwards. One could recommend increasing boluses by

50% for one to two days, 25% for one to two days, etc., but that requires the patient to either do the math, or reset all their rates more than once. It would be easier if a temporary bolus adjustment of 150% for 24–48 hours could be set, then another for 125% for 48 hours, and so on. It would also be helpful for regulating blood glucoses before menses, or lowering boluses at the end of the menses or with increased activity.

■ The ability to set correction (insulin sensitivity) factor([s] CF) by blood glucose levels instead of just by time of day. As glucose levels rise above 240–250 mg/dl, the amount of insulin needed to return the blood glucose to its target level may increase. For example, if a patient's CF is 40 (i.e., 1 unit decreases blood glucose about 40 mg/dl), when the patient's blood glucose is above 240 mg/dl, 1 unit of insulin may decrease the blood glucose level only 30 mg/dl.

■ Simpler pumps for type 2 patients, in whom carbohydrate counting does not need to be as precise. These could allow a pre-set breakfast, lunch, and dinner bolus, perhaps with sizes like small, medium, or large.

■ Glucose meters and glucose sensors that could connect via Bluetooth technology to one's car's system to alert the person to hypoglycemia and instruct the person to stop driving and treat the hypoglycemia. The global position system (GPS) could also indicate where the closest location is to purchase fruit juice or candy, if needed, with the hours of the establishment displayed. Even better would be a system that uses a GPS locator and enables a message with the glucose value and rate of change and the person's location to a designated person or list of people if the blood glucose dropped to a critical level (Wolfsdorf 2012). If the system were linked to an insulin pump, the system could automatically suspend the pump, decrease the basal rate, or stop a bolus in progress (such as an extended bolus) to prevent further hypoglycemia.

Great progress has been made, and continues to be made, with pump and sensor technology. We are closer to a "cure"—a viable closed-loop system. Until then, we hope this book helps the reader to successfully start patients on pump therapy, to make appropriate adjustments in followup, and troubleshoot common problems and challenges. We hope it helps you choose the right patient for a pump, the right pump for each patient, and the right settings for each patient's pump.

## REFERENCES

American Diabetes Association: Diabetic retinopathy. *Diabetes Care* 25 (Suppl 1):s90–s93, 2002

Blagg CR: The early history of dialysis for chronic renal failure in the United States: a view from Seattle. *Am J Kid Dis* 49:482–496, 2007

Bliss M: *The Discovery of Insulin.* Chicago: University of Chicago Press, 1982

Diabetes Control and Complications Research Group: The effect of intensive treatment of diabetes on the development and progression of long-term complications in insulin-dependent diabetes mellitus. *N Engl J Med* 329:977–986, 1993

Hirsch IB: Insulin analogues. *N Engl J Med* 352:174–183, 2005

King BR, Gross PW, Patterson MA, Crock PA, Anderson DG: Changes in altitude cause unintended insulin delivery from insulin pumps: mechanisms and implications. *Diabetes Care* 34:1932–1933, 2011

Mendosa D: History of blood glucose meters; transcripts of the interviews. http://www.mendosa.com/history.htm. Accessed 9 February 2013

Morris PJ: Transplantation: a medical miracle of the 20th century. *N Engl J Med* 351:2678–2680, 2004

Pickup JC, Keen H: Insulin pump therapy for type 1 diabetes. *N Engl J Med* 366:1616–1624, 2012

Wolfsdorf JI, ed: *Intensive Diabetes Management, 5th ed.* Alexandria, VA: American Diabetes Association, 2012

# Index

A1C targets, 33–34
Accessories
Active insulin (insulin on board), 93–94, 113–115
Adhesion, 95, 128–129, 211–212
Adolescents, teens, 157–158
Air bubbles/gaps, 99
Airports, air travel, 136–141
Alcohol, 108, 120–122
Amylin, 72–73
Apidra, 97
Attachments, 12–13

Babysitters, day care, 157
Backups, replacements, 16, 38, 100–103, 205–207, 218–219
Basal rates
adjustment, 86–92, 139–140
airports, air travel, 136–141
alternate, 90, 91
children, 154
exercise/sports, 89–91, 215, 217
factors affecting, 87–89, 91
insulin-resistance, 55
pattern establishment, 89–90
prolonged exercise, adjustment, 124
starting, determination of, 55–57
temporary, 90–92
tips, 215–216
tips for HCPs, 204
Bathing, showering, 42, 208
Batteries, 8, 12, 16, 20–21, 106, 209, 214, 218, 245
Binge eating, 141
Blood glucose
meter data usage, 84–85
postprandial, 33–34, 52, 55, 72, 74, 87–88, 113–119, 144, 148, 216–217
targets, 33–34, 52–54, 144, 148
target values determination, 33–34, 52–54
Blood in tubing, 100
Bolus calculators, 113–114

Bolus doses
adjustment, 114, 118–119
calculation, 36, 160–161
children, 155
compensatory, 130
exercise, hypoglycemia prevention, 122–124
extended/square wave, combination/dual wave, 117–119
meal bolus calculation, 62–64
missed, 120
postprandial, 113–119, 155, 216–217, 221
restaurants, dining out, 115–120
split, 72, 117
tips, 216–217
Buttonology, 6, 10, 41, 51, 90, 102, 152, 154–155, 204–205
Calculations
bolus doses, 36, 160–161
correction (sensitivity) factor, 62, 70, 93–94, 216
insulin-to-carbohydrate ratio, 58–61, 92–93, 216
meal bolus, 62–64
Carbohydrate counting, 35–37, 160–161
Case studies, 219–242
Children
adolescents, teens, 157–158
babies, toddlers, pre-school, 152–154
babysitters, day care, 157
basal rates, 154
blood glucose, A1C targets, 33–34, 148
bolus doses, 155
education of, 29
hypoglycemic unawareness, 147
insulin requirements in, 146–147
knowledge/skills by developmental age, 149–150
parents' roles, responsibilities, 151–152, 154–155, 158
patient selection, 24, 150–151
pump readiness determination, 147–152

pump selection, 11, 14–16
reverse dawn phenomenon, 147
school-aged, 155–157
type 1 diabetes, 157–159
Clocks, 12, 90
Communication between devices, 13
Continuous glucose monitor (CGM), 13, 35,
        72, 85–86
Correction (sensitivity) factor calculation, 62,
        70, 93–94, 216
Costs, 8, 20–21, 25
Customer service/technical support, 20–22,
        203–204, 207

Daily wear, 41–42, 95, 207–208
Dawn phenomenon, 87–88, 143
Day care, babysitters, 157
Dental surgery, 48, 105, 108, 132
Detemir, 143
Diabetes Medical Management Plan (DMMP),
        156
Diabulemia, 141
Dining out, restaurants, 115–120
Duration of insulin action feature, 93–94,
        113–115

East Virginia Medical Center, 145–146
Eating disorders, 141
Education. see patient education
Elderly patients, 162–163
Emergency care plans, 156
Emergency supplies, 100–103, 205–207,
        218–219
Ethnic foods, 115–120
Exercise
    basal rate changes, 89–91, 215,
        217
    delayed effects, 125
    hypoglycemia prevention, 122–124
    overview, 43, 122
    prolonged, basal adjustment, 124
    temperature extremes, 129
    tips, 215, 217
    troubleshooting, 104, 106, 108, 221
    wearing during, 127–129, 212
Exercise-induced hyperglycemia, 125–127

Food databases, 36
Forms
    Insulin Pump Therapy Evaluation, 172,
        174–175
    Insulin Pump Therapy Follow-Up, 172, 178
    Insulin Pump Therapy Information
        for Medical Procedure/
        Hospitalization/Surgery, 173,
        190–192
    Insulin Pump Therapy Physician Start
        Orders/Prescription, 172,
        176–177
    Insulin Pump Therapy Preparation
        Guidelines, 173, 184–185
    Insulin Pump Therapy Start Guidelines,
        173, 185–187
    Insulin Pump Therapy Telephone Follow-
        Up, 172, 180
    U-500 Regular Insulin Instructions/
        Information, 173, 193–195

Gastroparesis, 71–73, 109
Gestational diabetes, 162
Glargine, 143
Glucagon, 28, 38
Glucose meters, 244–245
Glulisine, 143

Hematomas, 98
Hibiclens, 98
History storage, 13, 16
Holiday foods, 115–120
Hormonal changes. see menstruation,
        hormone changes
Hospitalization
    forms, 173, 190–191
    preparations, 131–132, 145
Hyperglycemia
    algorithm correction, 65–67
    causes of, 6–7, 37–38, 214
    correction (sensitivity) factor calculation,
        62, 70, 93–94, 216
    exercise-induced, 125–127
    glucose sensor usage, 86
    inconsistent AM, 55–56
    insulin dosage correction, 65–66
    insulin leakage, 98–99

pattern management, 67–68
postprandial, 4, 72–73, 92, 115, 143
pregnancy, 144
prolonged exercise, basal adjustment, 124
pump troubleshooting, 64–65
troubleshooting, 103–106
Hypertension, 244
Hypoglycemia
    causes of, 86–87, 121
    delayed-onset, 125
    glucose sensor usage, 86
    identification of, 68
    insulin stacking, 15, 38, 66, 78, 86, 94, 107,
        114, 154
    management of, 68–69, 214–215
    pattern management, 6, 38–39
    postprandial, 66, 69, 93–94
    pramlintide, 3, 72–74
    prevention, 122–124
    troubleshooting, 69, 107–109
Hypoglycemia unawareness, 3, 147

Individualized Health Plan (IHP), 156
Infections, 7, 96, 98, 100
Infusion sets
    adhesion, 95, 128–129, 211–212
    daily wear, 41–42, 95, 207–209
    exercise, wearing during, 127–128
    features, 9–10
    insertion, removal, 29, 39–40, 98,
        211–213
    metal/steel needle, 17–19, 40, 100
    patch/pod, 9–10, 40
    proprietary, 17
    selection of, 16–20
    site rotation, 39–40, 96–97, 211–213
    skin irritation, 7, 40, 98
    Teflon cannula, 18–19, 40, 100
    tips, 210–213
    tubing (see tubing)
Infusion site infections, 7, 96, 98, 100
Inpatient admissions, 48
Insulin
    dosage correction, 65–66
    efficacy, 97
    history, 243–244
    leakage, 98–99

pens, 101, 103
pods, 9–10, 40, 96
stacking, 15, 38, 66, 78, 86, 94, 107, 114, 154
syringes, 101, 103, 243
U-500, 74–80, 159, 173, 193–195
Insulin on board (active insulin), 93–94,
    113–115
Insulin pump therapy. see also infusion sets;
    pumps
    benefits, 2–4
    challenges, 5–8
    described, 2
    indications for, 24
    myths, 4–5
    overview, 1–2
    pregnancy (see pregnancy)
Insulin-resistance
    insulin-to-carbohydrate ratio, 61
    medication adjustments, 162
    starting basal rate, 55
    U-500, 77–78, 159
Insulin-to-carbohydrate ratio calculation,
    58–61, 92–93, 216
Insurance, 7–8, 21–22, 25, 38, 44–45,
    151–152, 159

Ketoacidosis, 7, 101, 126, 144
Ketones, 38, 105, 108, 126
Ketone test strips, 38, 67, 103

Lancets, 244–245
Latent autoimmune diabetes in adulthood
    (LADA). see type 1.5 diabetes
Learning curve, 6
Lifestyle issues
    bathing, showering, 42, 208
    daily wear, 41–42, 95, 207–208
    medical procedures, 43, 48, 105, 108,
        130–133
    sexual activity, 43, 91, 129–130
    sick days, 43, 130–133
    sleeping, 42, 208
    sports, exercise (see exercise)
Lipohypertrophy, 39–40
Lispro, 118
Log books. see record keeping
Logistics/placement, 7, 12, 39–40

Meal bolus calculation, 62–64
Medical identification, 39
Medical procedures
    forms, 173, 191–192
    preparations, 43, 48, 105, 108, 130–133
Medicare, 20–21, 25–26, 159
Medication changes, 105, 108, 161–162
Menopause, 105, 108, 142
Menstruation, hormone changes
    basal rate changes, 48, 89–90, 215
    hyperglycemia/hypoglycemia, 38, 91, 105,
        108
    pump usage generally, 142
    record keeping, 70, 83–84
Multiple daily injection (MDI), 1, 3, 24, 41

NovoLog, 97

Patient education
    basal rate delivery, 14 (see also basal rates)
    bolus delivery, 15 (see also bolus doses)
    buttonology, 6, 10, 41, 51, 90, 102, 152,
        154–155, 204–205
    criteria checklist, 11–13
    goals, objectives, 31–35
    initiation of therapy, 22
    insulin, insulin delivery, 13–14
    overview, 10–11
    pump start-up (see pump start-up)
    safety, 15–16
    steps, methods, 28–30
    tips for HCPs, 204–205
Patient selection
    contraindications, 27–28
    profile, 23–27, 37
    tips for HCPs, 205
Pediatrics. see children
Perimenopause, 105, 108, 142
Pets, 101, 213
Physical activity. see exercise
Pizza, 118
Pramlintide, 3, 72–74, 107
Pregestational diabetes, 143, 145
Pregnancy
    gestational diabetes, 162
    glucose control, recommended targets,
        144

    hyperglycemia, 144 (see also
        hyperglycemia)
    labor, C section, 145–146
    medicines contraindicated, 73
    post-delivery insulin needs, 146
    pregestational diabetes, 143, 145
    pump benefits, 4, 144
    pump usage during, 142–146
    type 2 diabetes, 162
Pump bumps, 98
Pump clocks, 12, 90
Pumps
    basal rate delivery, 14
    bolus calculators, 113–114
    bolus delivery, 15 (see also bolus dose)
    criteria checklist, 11–13
    features, 9–10
    features in development, 246–248
    history of, 245
    insulin, insulin delivery, 13–14
    insulin on board (active insulin), 93–94,
        113–115
    orders, initial, 45–46, 50
    patch type, 10
    pod type, 10
    safety, 15–16
    selection of, 10–11
    start-up (see pump start-up)
    state of the art, 245–246
    therapy management (see therapy
        management)
    troubleshooting, 64–65
    tubing (see tubing)
    waterproof, water-resistant, 128
Pump start-up
    appointment schedules, 71
    blood glucose target values determination,
        33–34, 52–54
    clinician guidelines, 50–52
    correction (sensitivity) factor calculation,
        62, 70, 93–94, 216
    dietary adjustments, 70
    exercise, 70
    follow-up, 69–71
    hyperglycemia (see hyperglycemia)
    hypoglycemia (see hypoglycemia)
    insulin dosages, 49

insulin-to-carbohydrate ratio calculation, 58–61, 92–93, 216

    meal bolus calculation, 62–64

    overview, 31

    patient guidelines, 49–50

    priming tips, 210

    responsibilities, 47–49

    SMBG, 69–70

    starting basal determination (see basal rates)

Rapid-acting insulin analogs, 101, 114, 144

Record keeping

    forms, 173, 179, 181, 188–189

    log book, 70, 83–84

    tips, 214

Reservoir (see Cartridge/reservoir)

Resources

    accessories, 197

    books, 33, 36, 197–198

    Fact Sheet—Air Travel and Diabetes, 138

    federal laws, school responsibilities, 156

    forms (see forms)

    Internet, 44, 152, 200–201

    magazines, 198–199

    manufacturers, 196–197

    organizations, associations, 199–200

    support groups, 29–30, 32

    TSA Cares Help Line, 136

Restaurants, dining out, 115–120

Reverse dawn phenomenon, 147

Rule of 15, 38, 104, 214–215, 221

Saline trials, 41

School-aged children, 155–157

Selection

    of infusion sets, 16–20

    patient (see patient selection)

    of pumps, 10–11

Self-monitoring of blood glucose (SMBG)

    CGM data usage, 85–86

    frequency of, 34

    necessity of, 2, 6

    pump start-up, 69–70

Sensitivity (correction) factor calculation, 62, 70, 93–94, 216

Sexual activity, 43, 91, 129, 130

Shipping, 22

Showering, bathing, 42, 208

Sick days, 43, 130–133

Site rotation, 39–40, 96–97, 211–213

Skin irritation, 7, 40, 98

Sleep apnea

Sleeping, 42, 208

Smartphones, 36

Smart pumps, 35, 70, 84

Spandex, 128

Special meals, 115–120

Special-needs patients, 162–163

SportPak, 128

Stacking insulin, 15, 38, 66, 78, 86, 94, 107, 114, 154

Staphylococcus, 98, 100

Stress (emotional)

    basal rate changes, 48, 89–90, 215

    hyperglycemia/hypoglycemia, 38, 91, 105, 108

    pump usage generally, 133–134

    record keeping, 70, 83–84

Supplies

    carrying, tips, 218–219

    emergency, 100–103, 205–207, 218–219

    hospitalization, 131–132

    ordering, 20, 44–46

Support

    of children, 151–152, 154–155, 158

    family/friends, 44, 71

    groups, 29–30, 32

    resources (see resources)

    technical, 20–22, 203–204, 207

Surgery

    forms, 173, 190–192

    preparations, 43, 48, 105, 108, 130–133

Technical support, 20–22, 203–204, 207

Therapy management

    basal rates (see basal rates)

    blood glucose meter data usage, 84–85

    CGM data usage, 85–86

    data usage, 84

    explanations, 83

    healthcare practitioners in, 30, 113

    insulin on board (active insulin), 93–94, 113–115

pump clocks, 12, 90
record keeping (log book), 70, 83–84
Thinkpads, 36
Tips
    basal rates, 215–216
    batteries, 8, 12, 16, 20–21, 106, 209, 214, 218, 245
    bolus doses, 216–217
    cartridge/reservoir, 209–210
    exercise/sports, 215, 217
    general for patients, 206–207
    for HCPs, 203–206
    infusion sets, 210–213
    priming, 210
    pump settings, 213–215
    supplies, carrying, 218–219
    wearing options, 207–208
Traveling, 134–140, 215
Troubleshooting
    exercise, 104, 106, 108, 221
    hyperglycemia, 103–106
    hypoglycemia, 69, 107–109
    insulin stacking, 15, 38, 66, 78, 86, 94, 107, 114, 154
    pumps, 64–65
    tubing, 106
TSA Cares Help Line, 136
TSA guidelines, 136–138
Tubing
    air bubbles/gaps, 99
    blood in, 100
    changing, 97
    infusion sets, 16–20, 97, 154–155
    insulin leakage, 98–99
    pumps, 13–14
    tips, 210–213
    troubleshooting, 106
Type 1 diabetes
    alcohol, 121
    benefits of pump therapy, 2–3
    case studies, 219–242
    children, 157–159
    exercise benefits, 122
    follow-up visits, 71
    gastroparesis, 71–73, 109
    history, 116, 243–245

hypoglycemia (see hypoglycemia)
hypoglycemia unawareness, 121
ketones, 38, 105, 108, 126
meal boluses, 116–117
medical procedures (see medical procedures)
Medicare, 25–26
menarche/menopause/menstruation, 142
plasma blood glucose/A1C goals, 34, 148
pramlintide, 3, 72–74, 107
pregnancy, delivery, 146
pump initiation (see pump start-up)
starting basal rate determination, 55–57
weight changes, 6, 140–141
Type 1.5 diabetes, 26, 158–161
Type 2 diabetes
    benefits, 3–4, 158–161
    bolus dose calculation, 36, 160–161
    contraindications, 160
    hypoglycemia (see hypoglycemia)
    Medicare, 25–26
    medication adjustments, 105, 108, 161–162
    pramlintide, 3, 72–74, 107
    pregnancy, 162
    pump initiation (see pump start-up)
    pump selection, 11
    sleep apnea in, 55
    U-500, 74–80, 159, 173, 193–195

U-500
    forms, 173, 193–195
    overview, 74–80, 159
Untethered programs, 127
User's manuals, 51, 185–187, 204, 206–207

Warranties, 20–21, 50, 51
Wear, daily, 41–42, 95, 207–208
Weight changes, 6, 140–141

Zipps, 128

CPSIA information can be obtained
at www.ICGtesting.com
Printed in the USA
FSHW021436040320
67805FS